Periodontal Disease
- Diagnostic and
Adjunctive Non-surgical
Considerations

Edited by
Nermin Mohammed Ahmed Yussif

Published in London, United Kingdom

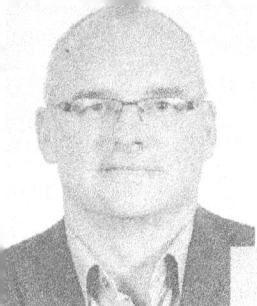
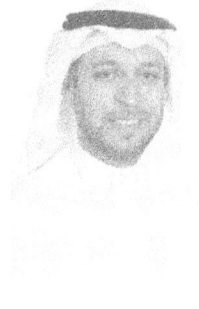
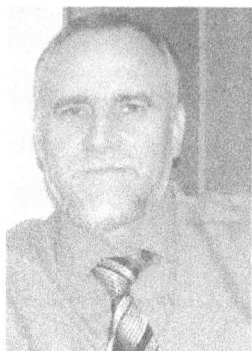
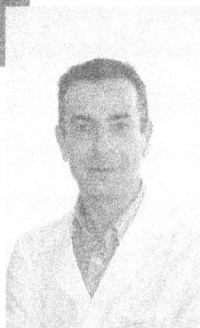
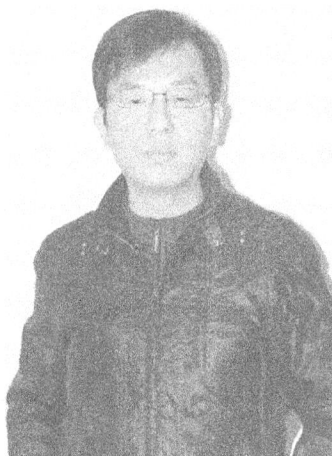
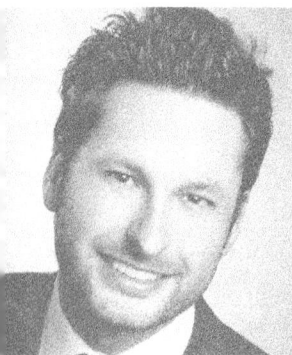
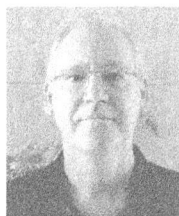

IntechOpen

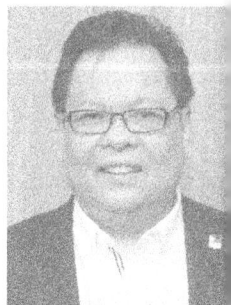
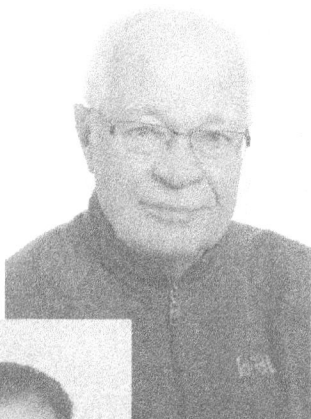
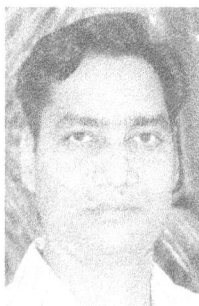
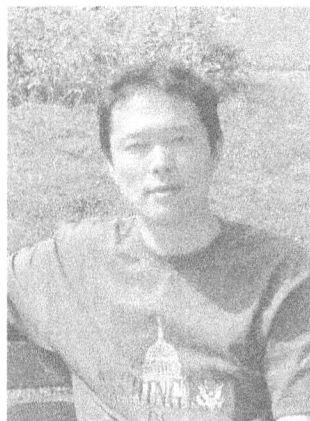
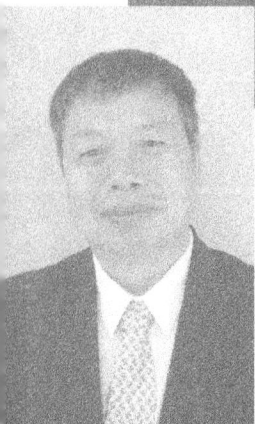
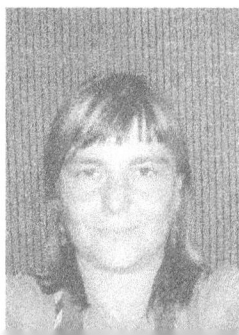

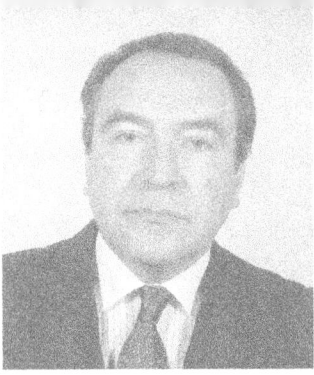

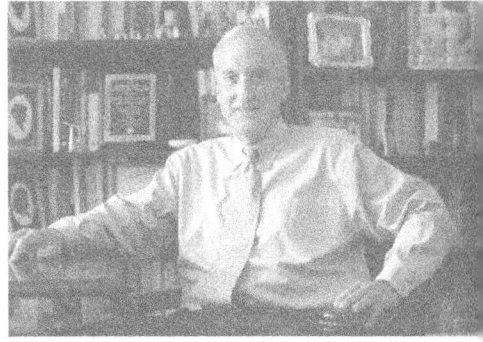

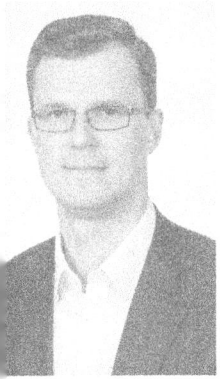

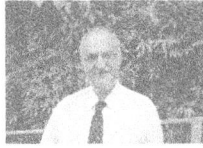

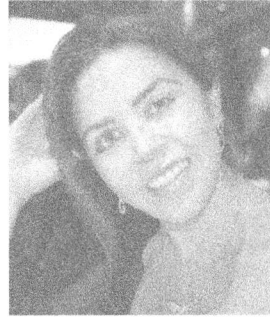

Supporting open minds since 2005

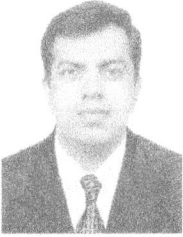

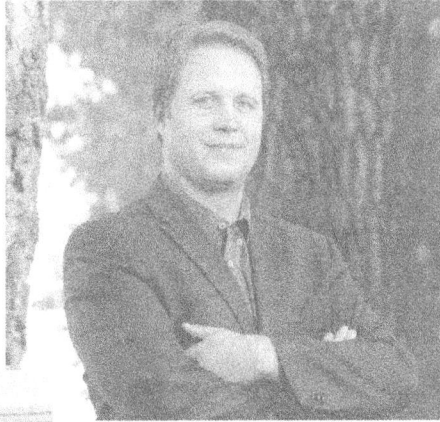

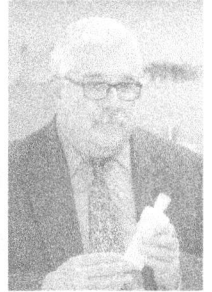

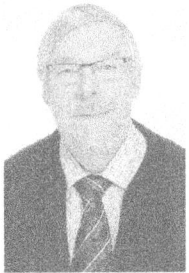

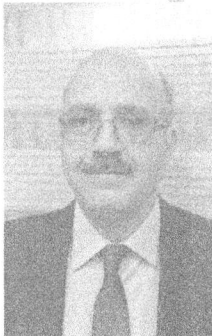

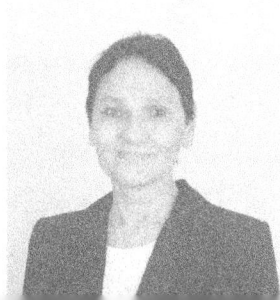

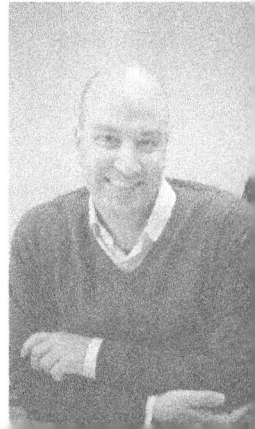

Periodontal Disease - Diagnostic and Adjunctive Non-surgical Considerations
http://dx.doi.org/10.5772/intechopen.78158
Edited by Nermin Mohammed Ahmed Yussif

Part of IntechOpen Book Series: Dentistry, Volume 6
Book Series Editor: Zühre Akarslan

Contributors
Gurumoorthy Kaarthikeyan, Swarna Meenakshi, Nermin Mohammed Ahmed Yussif, Javier González-Ramírez, Nicolas Serafin-Higuera, Gustavo Martínez-Coronilla, Silva-Mancilla Marina Concepción, Ana Laura López-López, Jesus Famania-Bustamante, Krishna Kripal, Aiswarya Dileep, Jose Luis Muñoz-Carrillo, Viridiana Elizabeth Hernández-Reyes, Francisca Chávez Ruvalcaba, María Isabel Chávez Ruvalcaba, Karla Mariana Chávez Ruvalcaba, Lizbeth Díaz Alfaro, Oscar Eduardo García Huerta

Notice
Statements and opinions expressed in the chapters are these of the individual contributors and not necessarily those of the editors or publisher. No responsibility is accepted for the accuracy of information contained in the published chapters. The publisher assumes no responsibility for any damage or injury to persons or property arising out of the use of any materials, instructions, methods or ideas contained in the book.

First published in London, United Kingdom, 2020 by IntechOpen
IntechOpen is the global imprint of INTECHOPEN LIMITED, registered in England and Wales, registration number: 11086078, 7th floor, 10 Lower Thames Street, London, EC3R 6AF, United Kingdom
Printed in Croatia

British Library Cataloguing-in-Publication Data
A catalogue record for this book is available from the British Library

Additional hard and PDF copies can be obtained from orders@intechopen.com

Periodontal Disease - Diagnostic and Adjunctive Non-surgical Considerations
Edited by Nermin Mohammed Ahmed Yussif
p. cm.
Print ISBN 978-1-78984-460-3
Online ISBN 978-1-78984-461-0
eBook (PDF) ISBN 978-1-83880-136-6
ISSN 2631-6218

We are IntechOpen,
the world's leading publisher of
Open Access books
Built by scientists, for scientists

4,600+
Open access books available

119,000+
International authors and editors

135M+
Downloads

Our authors are among the

151
Countries delivered to

Top 1%
most cited scientists

12.2%
Contributors from top 500 universities

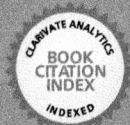

Interested in publishing with us?
Contact book.department@intechopen.com

Numbers displayed above are based on latest data collected.
For more information visit www.intechopen.com

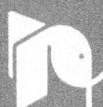

IntechOpen Book Series

Dentistry

Volume 6

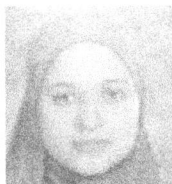

Nermin Yussif received her MSc degree in dental laserology (2013), her MSc degree in periodontology, and her PhD degree in periodontology (2019), all from the University of Cairo (Egypt). Her first training as general practitioner was in Kasr El Aini Hospital, Faculty of Dentistry, Cairo University. Her research journey began in 2009 in the National Institute of Laser Sciences, Cairo University, Egypt. She is currently a lecturer and researcher in the Faculty of Dentistry, Cairo University. Her current research interests and expertise include periodontology, periodontal plastic surgeries, dental laserology, oral implantology, oral mesotherapy, nutrition for therapeutic purposes, and dental pharmacotherapy.

Editor of Volume 6: Nermin Yussif
Periodontology department- Faculty of Dentistry, MSA University, Giza, Egypt
MSc-Dental laser applications- NILES, Cairo University, Egypt

Series Editor: Zühre Akarslan
Gazi University Faculty of Dentistry, Turkey

Scope of the Series

The major pathologies which dentists encounter in clinical practice include dental caries and periodontal diseases. Diagnosis and treatment of these pathologies is essential because when untreated, abscess could occur and it can even lead to the extraction of the tooth. Extracted teeth can be replaced with implants. Dentists and patients are nowadays more familiar with dental implant treatments. As a result, advanced diagnostic tools which aid in pre-operative treatment planning (cone-beam computed tomography, computer aided implant planning etc..), new implant designs improving the success of osteointegration, new materials, and techniques are introduced in the dental market.

Conditions which dentists frequently encounter in their clinical practice are temporomandibular joint (TMJ) disorders. These disorders include degenerative musculoskeletal conditions associated with morphological and functional deformities. Accurate diagnosis is important for proper management of TMJ pathologies. With the advance in technology, new materials, techniques and equipment are introduced in the dental practice. New diagnostic aids in dental caries detection, cone-beam computed tomographic imaging, soft and hard tissue lasers, advances in oral and maxillofacial surgery procedures, uses of ultrasound, CAD/CAM, nanotechnology, plasma rich protein (PRP) and dental implantology are some of them. There will be even more new applications in dentistry in the future.

This book series includes topics related to dental caries, dentomaxillofacial imaging, new trends in oral implantology, new approaches in oral and maxillofacial surgery, temporomandibular joint disorders in dentistry etc.

Contents

Preface

Periodontal diseases are a group of chronic immune-inflammatory diseases that, according to their severity, may induce different levels of periodontal destruction. Such diseases could range from mild gingivitis to severe periodontitis. Although there is similarity in the nature of the periodontal diseases in general, each disease has special characteristics. These characters could differ if the disease is solitary or it could be a reflection of a systemic disease.

The goal of this book is to clarify the main structure of periodontal diagnosis and discuss the most recent modalities in non-surgical adjunctive therapeutic aids.

Unfortunately, in 2019, periodontal diseases became some of the most common diseases that affect human beings all over the world. Periodontal diseases reported relatively higher prevalence in developing countries, especially in children due to nutrition deficiency, hygiene problems, awareness, low educational and social levels, limited financial aids, and limited diagnostic privilege.

The multifactorial nature of the disease makes the early identification and diagnosis more difficult. Therefore, it is clear that there is no single diagnostic aid that can provide full clinical assessment of the different periodontal conditions.

The higher prevalence of periodontal diseases is mainly due to the delay of the patients asking for dental examination and treatment at the onset stage of the disease. Unfortunately, patients usually ask for diagnosis and treatment when the disease reaches an advanced stage. Late diagnosis could lead to loss of the affected teeth as well as severe damage to the remaining structures. Nowadays, there is great improvement in the diagnostic aids that could facilitate the early discovery of such diseases.

The main requirements that are needed for an ideal diagnostic aid is to be easy to use, informative, non-invasive, cost effective, and accepted by patients. Nowadays, biomarkers, radiographic evaluations, and genetic analysis are the main informative and most recent diagnostic aids in the periodontal field.

In the last few decades, biomarkers have developed great potential to be used for diagnosis of periodontal diseases. The main function of the biomarker is to indicate the presence and severity of the disease and report the responses of the periodontal tissues to any therapeutic interventions.

The great evolution in the radiographic aids makes the early monitoring of the changes of periodontal hard structure easier. There has been development of a wide spectrum of radiographic techniques such as the subtractive and topographic technique.

Lately, the literature has recorded several non-surgical techniques that could act as adjunctive modalities to treat mild to moderate conditions and serve as a treatment aid in severe conditions. LASER therapy, photodynamic therapy, oral mesotherapy, and locally delivered antibiotics and anti-inflammatories are all examples of this.

Hopefully, this book will serve as a guide and an overview for researchers and practitioners who are interested in the periodontal diagnosis and non-surgical therapeutic modalities. I really hope this book could inspire researchers for future research and innovative ideas. The book consists of six chapters, with each chapter focussing on a certain point of the diagnostic aids. All chapters attempt to cover the topic in a systematic way starting with background information on the subject, with a detailed description for the advantages, limitations, types, methods to apply the technique, and points of future research.

Chapter 1 describes an overview of the pathogenesis of periodontal diseases and the contributing factors in periodontal destruction. **Chapter 2** describes in-depth the role of biomarkers in diagnosis of periodontal diseases. The advantages and limitations of the various biomarkers will be discussed in order to recognize new points of research. In **Chapter 3**, the genetic biomarkers are discussed to clarify the role of the diagnostic aids in specifying the association between the periodontal disease and genetic disorders such as gene polymorphism. **Chapter 4** gives a detailed description about the role of the radiographic revolution as a diagnostic aid for periodontal diseases. In **Chapter 5**, an overview of one of the most recent non-surgical adjunctive modalities, oral mesotherapy, is presented. This technique provides promising results in the management of periodontal diseases and is considered as a virgin point for future research.

Nermin Mohammed Ahmed Yussif
Periodontology Department - Faculty of Dentistry,
MSA University,
Giza, Egypt

MSc - Dental Laser Applications - NILES,
Cairo University,
Egypt

Section 1

Pathogenesis of Periodontal Diseases

Chapter 1

Pathogenesis of Periodontal Disease

José Luis Muñoz-Carrillo, Viridiana Elizabeth Hernández-Reyes,
Oscar Eduardo García-Huerta, Francisca Chávez-Ruvalcaba,
María Isabel Chávez-Ruvalcaba, Karla Mariana Chávez-Ruvalcaba
and Lizbeth Díaz-Alfaro

Abstract

Inflammation is a physiological response of the innate immune system against several endogenous or exogenous stimuli. Inflammation begins with an acute pattern; however, it can become chronic by activating the adaptive immune response through cellular and noncellular mechanisms. The main etiologic factor of periodontal disease is bacteria which substantially harbor the human oral cavity. The most common periodontal diseases are gingivitis and periodontitis, whose main characteristic is inflammation. The knowledge of how immune mechanisms and inflammatory responses are regulated is fundamental to understanding the pathogenesis of periodontal disease. The purpose of this chapter is to show the current panorama of the immunological mechanisms involved in the pathogenesis of periodontal disease.

Keywords: periodontal tissues, biofilm, inflammatory response, innate and adaptive immunity, periodontitis

1. Introduction

Periodontitis is a globally widespread pathology of the human oral cavity. Approximately 10% of the global adult population is highly vulnerable to severe periodontitis, and 10–15% appears to be completely resistant to it, while the remainder varies between these two situations [1]. Periodontitis is a major public health problem due to its high prevalence, as well as because it may lead to tooth loss and disability, negatively affect chewing function and aesthetics, be a source of social inequality, and impair the quality of life. Periodontitis accounts for a substantial proportion of edentulism and masticatory dysfunction, results in significant dental care costs, and has a plausible negative impact on general health [2].

2. Periodontal support tissues

The periodontium is a complex of tissues with blood vessels, nerves, and bundles of fibers, which provide nutrition and sensibility, supporting and investing the tooth. The periodontium has the potential for regeneration and remodeling throughout life, which allows the primary dentition to be transient and to be replaced by the permanent dentition [3, 4]. It is important to understand that each of the periodontal tissues has a very specialized structure and that these structural characteristics directly define the function. In fact, the proper functioning of the periodontium is only achieved through the structural integrity and interaction between its components [4].

The periodontium is one of the morphofunctional components of the stomato-gnathic system, and its "design" not only responds to intrinsic functions related to nutrition or the subjection of the tooth but also to functions integrated within the physiology of the stomatognathic system [5]. The main function of the periodon-tium is to join the tooth to the bone tissue and maintain integrity on the surface of the masticatory mucosa of the oral cavity [6]. The periodontium includes four tissues located near the teeth: (1) the alveolar bone (AB), (2) root cementum (CR), (3) periodontal ligament (PL), and (4) gingiva (G) (e.g., **Figure 1a**) [4, 7, 8].

2.1 Alveolar bone

The alveolar bone, together with the root cementum and the periodontal ligament, constitutes the tooth insertion apparatus, whose main function is to distribute the forces generated by chewing and other contacts [6]. The maxilla and mandible of the adult human can be subdivided into two parts: (a) the alveolar process that involves in housing the roots of the erupted teeth and (b) the basal body that does not involve in housing the roots [8].

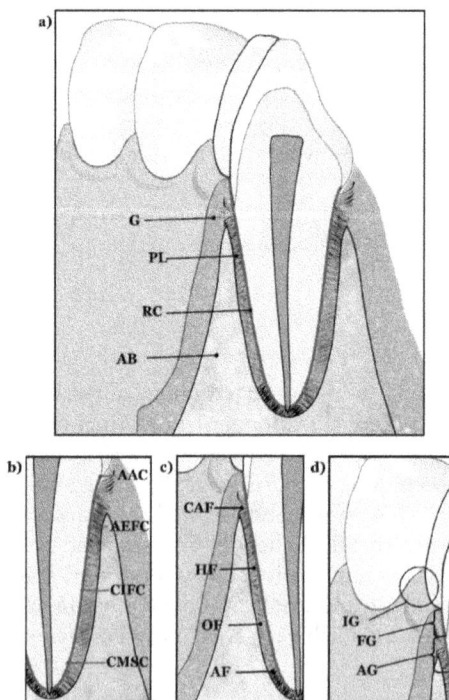

Figure 1.
Periodontal tissues. (a) Tissues that support the tooth include the alveolar bone (AB), root cementum (RC), periodontal ligament (PL), and gingiva (G). (b) Forms of cementum: acellular afibrillar cementum (AAC), acellular extrinsic fibers cementum (AEFC), cellular mixed stratified cementum (CMSC), and cellular intrinsic fibers cementum (CIFC). (c) Bundles of collagen fibers: crestal alveolar fibers (CAF), horizontal fibers (HF), oblique fibers (OF), and apical fibers (AF). (d) Parts of the gingiva: free gingiva (FG), interdental gingiva (IG), and attached gingiva (AG).

The alveolar process is the bone of the jaws that contain the sockets (alveoli) of the teeth. It consists of outer cortical plates (buccal, lingual, and palatal) of the compact bone, a central spongiosa, and bone lining the alveolus (alveolar bone) [4]. The alveolar process is dependent on the teeth as they develop and remodel with their formation and eruption. Therefore, the shape, location, and function of the teeth determine its morphology [8]. The periodontal ligament contains progenitor cells that can differentiate into osteoblasts for the maintenance and repair of the alveolar bone. However, in the absence of the tooth, it is lost. These characteristics suggest that the regulatory mechanisms are important for the alveolar bone, so there is an interdependence of the periodontal tissues, which work together as a unit [4].

2.2 Root cementum

The root cementum is an avascular mineralized connective tissue covering the entire root surface, forming the interface between the root dentine and the periodontal ligament [6, 7]. In addition, the root cementum plays important roles in nourishing the tooth as well as in stabilizing the tooth via the attachment to the periodontal ligament. This enables the tooth to maintain its relationship to adjacent and opposing teeth [3]. Unlike the bone, the root cementum does not contain blood or lymphatic vessels, lacks innervation, and does not undergo remodeling or physiological resorption, but it is characterized by the fact that continues to be deposited throughout life [6]. The composition of cementum contains about 50% mineral (substituted apatite) and 50% organic matrix. Type I collagen is the predominant organic component, constituting up to 90% of the organic matrix. Other collagens associated with cementum include type I, III, V, VI, XII, and XIV [4].

Cementum performs different functions: it fixes the main fibers of the periodontal ligament to the root and contributes in the repair process when the root surface has been damaged [6]. Cementum has been classified as cellular and acellular cementum depending on the presence and absence of cementocytes, further grouped into intrinsic and extrinsic fiber cementum depending on the presence of collagen fibers formed by cementoblasts or by fibroblasts, respectively [8]. There are different forms of cementum (e.g., **Figure 1b**): (1) acellular afibrillar cementum (AAC), (2) acellular extrinsic fiber cementum (AEFC), (3) cellular mixed stratified cementum (CMSC), and (4) cellular intrinsic fibers cementum (CIFC) [4, 6].

2.3 Periodontal ligament

The periodontal ligament is the soft and specialized connective tissue situated between the cementum covering the root of the tooth and the bone forming the socket wall (alveolodental ligament) [4]. The periodontal ligament consists of cells and an extracellular compartment comprising collagenous and noncollagenous matrix constituents. The cells include osteoblasts and osteoclasts, fibroblasts, epithelial cell rests of Malassez, monocytes and macrophages, undifferentiated mesenchymal cells, and cementoblasts and odontoclasts. The extracellular compartment consists mainly of well-defined collagen fiber bundles embedded in an amorphous background material, known as ground substance [4, 8]. These bundles of collagen fibers can be classified into the following groups, according to their disposition (e.g., **Figure 1c**): crestal alveolar fibers (CAF), horizontal fibers (HF), oblique fibers (OF), and apical fibers (AF) [6].

The main function of the periodontal ligament is to support the teeth in their sockets and at the same time allow them to withstand the considerable forces of mastication. In addition, the periodontal ligament has the capacity to act as a sensory receptor necessary for the proper positioning of the jaws during mastication, and, very importantly, it is a cell reservoir for tissue homeostasis, regeneration, and repair [4].

2.4 Gingiva

Gingiva is a portion of the oral mucosa covering the tooth-carrying part of the alveolar bone and the cervical neck of the tooth. Three parts of the gingiva can be distinguished (e.g., **Figure 1d**): (1) free gingiva (FG), (2) interdental gingiva (IG), and (3) attached or inserted gingiva (AG) [6]. Histologically, the epithelial component of the gingiva shows regional morphological variations that reflect the adaptation of the tissue to the tooth and alveolar bone. These include the epithelium that covers a connective tissue, chorion, or lamina propria. A keratinized stratified squamous epithelium protects the lamina propria of the gingiva on its masticatory surfaces and a nonkeratinized epithelium protects the lamina propria on its crevicular and junctional surfaces [6, 9]. The junctional epithelium plays a crucial role since it essentially seals off periodontal tissues from the oral environment. Its integrity is thus essential for maintaining a healthy periodontium. Periodontal disease sets in when the structure of the junctional epithelium starts to fail, an excellent example of how structure determines function [4].

During pathological conditions, such as inflammation, the periodontal connective tissues, including the gingiva, undergo many changes. Clinically detected gingival overgrowth is one of the alterations that occurs in chronic periodontitis. It is caused by a variety of etiological factors and is exacerbated by local bacterial biofilm accumulation, because the periodontopathogen products act on the gingival tissues activating cellular events that induce the alteration of connective tissue homeostasis and the destruction of the alveolar bone [9]. Likewise, junctional epithelial cells differ considerably from those of the gingival epithelium. There are polymorphonuclear leukocytes and monocytes that pass from the subepithelial connective tissue through the junctional epithelium and into the gingival sulcus. The mononuclear cells, together with molecules they secrete and others originating from junctional epithelial cells, blood and tissue fluid, represent the first line of defense in the control of the perpetual microbial challenge [4].

3. Periodontal pathogenesis

Periodontitis is a chronic multifactorial disease characterized by an inflammation of the periodontal tissue mediated by the host, which is associated with dysbiotic plaque biofilms, resulting in the progressive destruction of the tooth-supporting apparatus and loss of periodontal attachment [1, 10]. The bacterial biofilm formation initiates gingival inflammation; however, periodontitis initiation and progression depend on dysbiotic ecological changes in the microbiome in response to nutrients from gingival inflammatory and tissue breakdown products and anti-bacterial mechanisms that attempt to contain the microbial challenge within the gingival sulcus area once inflammation has initiated. This leads to the activation of several key molecular pathways, which ultimately activate host-derived proteinases that enable loss of marginal periodontal ligament fibers, apical migration of the junctional epithelium, and allows apical spread of the bacterial biofilm along the root surface [1]. Therefore, the primary features of periodontitis include the loss of periodontal tissue support, manifested through clinical attachment loss and radiographically assessed alveolar bone loss, presence of periodontal pocketing, and gingival bleeding [10].

3.1 Periodontal histopathology

The development of gingivitis and periodontitis can be divided into a series of stages: initial, early, established, and advanced lesions (e.g., **Figure 2**) [11, 12]. The initial lesion begins 2–4 days after the accumulation of the microbial plaque. During the initial lesion, an acute exudative vasculitis in the plexus of the venules lateral to the junctional epithelium, migration of polymorphonuclear (PMN) cells through the junctional epithelium into the gingival sulcus, co-exudation of fluid from the sulcus, and the loss of perivascular collagen were observed. The early injury develops within 4–10 days. This lesion is characterized by a dense infiltrate of T lymphocytes and other mononuclear cells, as well as by the pathological alteration of the fibroblasts [6, 11–13].

Subsequently, the established lesion develops within 2–3 weeks. This lesion is dominated by activated B cells (plasma cells) and accompanied by further loss of the marginal gingival connective tissue matrix, but no bone loss is yet detectable. Several PMN continue to migrate through the junctional epithelium, and the gingival pocket is gradually established. Finally, in the advanced lesion, plasma cells continue to predominate as the architecture of the gingival tissue is disturbed, together with the destruction of the alveolar bone and periodontal ligament. It is characterized by a conversion of junctional epithelium to the pocket epithelium, formation of denser inflammatory infiltrate composed of plasma cells and macrophages, loss of collagen attachment to the root surface, and resorption of the alveolar bone [6, 11–13].

3.2 Immune responses in the pathogenesis of periodontal disease

In normal health conditions, periodontal tissues are capable of coping with the presence of bacteria through several mechanisms of the host immune system (e.g., **Figure 3**) [14]. However, when the balance between the infection control mechanisms and the subgingival biofilm is lost [15], which includes *Porphyromonas*

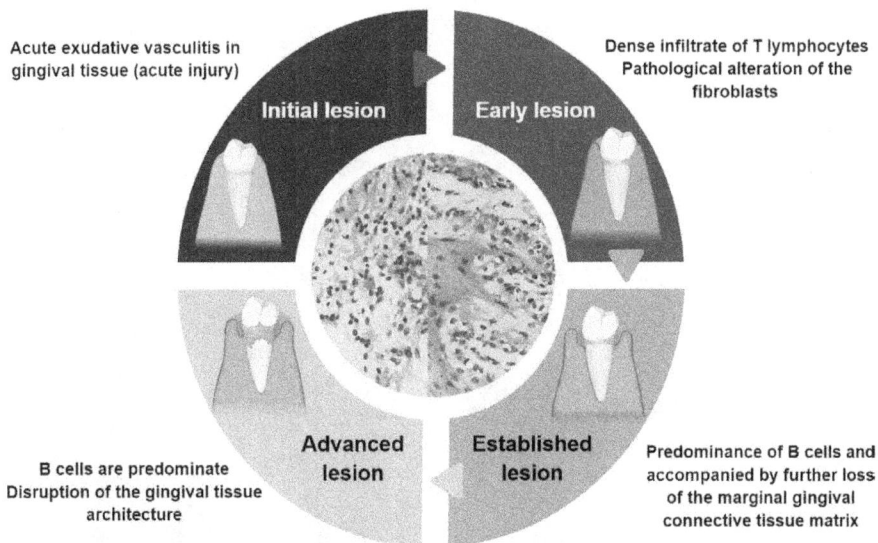

Figure 2.
Histopathological lesions of periodontal pathogenesis. Initial, early, established, and advanced lesions of the development of gingivitis and periodontitis.

gingivalis, *Aggregatibacter actinomycetemcomitans*, *Tannerella forsythia*, and *Treponema denticola* [16], innate, inflammatory, and adaptive reactions are triggered. These processes result in the destruction of the tissues that surround and support the teeth, and eventually in the loss of tissues, bones and finally, of the teeth [17].

3.2.1 Innate immune response in periodontal disease

The most important characteristic of periodontitis is the inflammatory reabsorption of the tooth-supporting alveolar bone due to the uncontrolled host immune response against periodontal infection, since the destructive events, which lead to the irreversible phenotype of periodontal disease, are the result of the persistence of a chronic and exacerbated inflammatory immune response [18]. Inflammation is a process of the innate immune system activation, in response to exogenous and endogenous factors, such as infection by microorganisms, tissue stress, and injuries. Inflammation is a protective response, characterized by its cardinal signs, such as redness, swelling, heat, pain, and disrupted function [19]. The inflammatory response consists of four main components: (1) endogenous or exogenous factors, such as molecular patterns associated with pathogens (PAMP) and damage (DAMP), which are derived from bacteria, viruses, fungi, parasites, and cell damage, as well as toxic cellular components or any other harmful condition; (2) cellular receptors that recognize these molecular patterns (PRR), for example, Toll-like receptors (TLR); (3) proinflammatory mediators, such as cytokines, chemokines, the complement system, etc.; and (4) target cells and tissues, where these proinflammatory mediators act [20, 21]. The inflammatory response is mainly characterized by four successive phases: (1) silent phase, where the cells synthesize and release the first proinflammatory mediators; (2) vascular phase, characterized by an increase in vascular permeability and dilatation; (3) cellular

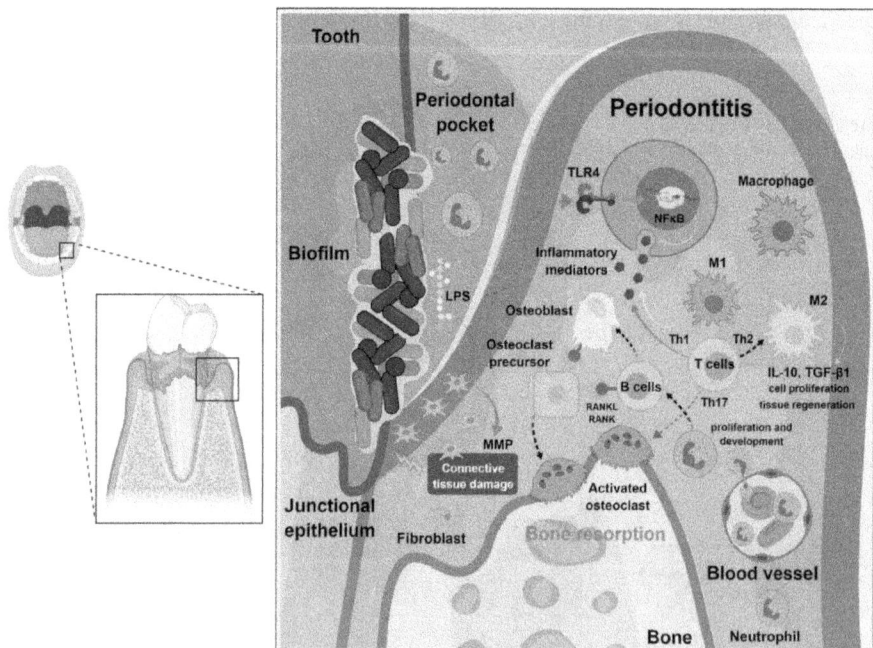

Figure 3.
Innate and adaptive immune response during periodontal disease (description in the text).

phase, characterized by the infiltration of inflammatory cells at the site of injury; and (4) the resolution of the inflammatory response [22].

The inflammatory immune response is triggered by the interaction of resident cells with the bacterial biofilm attached to the tooth surface. Bacterial biofilm attaches to the tooth surface, making it impossible for the immune system to eradicate the infecting microorganisms efficiently, perpetuating the insult to the periodontal tissues [18]. The junctional epithelium is the first periodontal structure to face the bacterial challenge [23]. Bacteria are capable to cross the junctional epithelium and pass to the gingival conjunctive tissue, where they stimulate the gingival epithelial cells and fibroblasts to trigger the initial inflammatory responses [24]. These resident periodontal cells detect bacterial PAMP, such as lipopolysaccharide (LPS) [25], which binds to the Toll-like receptors (TLR4/2), triggering the recruitment of several protein kinases in the cytoplasmic end of the receptors, ultimately causing the activation of proinflammatory transcription factors, such as nuclear factor kappa B (NFκB) and activator protein 1 (AP-1) [26], which induces the synthesis and release of mediators to trigger the inflammatory response. Likewise, the gingival fibroblasts and the periodontal ligament are responsible for the destruction and disorganization of the fibrous component of the extracellular matrix of the periodontal tissue by increasing the local production and the activity of the matrix metalloproteinases (MMPs) [27, 28].

The periodontal lesion is initiated as acute inflammation characterized by increased numbers of neutrophils migrating into the gingival crevice through the junctional epithelium, which have the de novo biosynthetic capacity for chemokines and cytokines with proinflammatory, anti-inflammatory, or immunoregulatory properties. Neutrophils, through the release of chemokines, can induce the recruitment of interleukin-17-producing CD4-positive T-helper 17 cells to sites of infection or inflammation. In addition, they can promote the survival, proliferation, and development of B cells into antibody-secreting plasma cells. Likewise, it was shown that activated neutrophils express membrane-bound receptor activator of nuclear factor kappa B ligand (RANKL), a key osteoclastogenic cytokine and, thereby able of inducing osteoclastic bone resorption [29]. These recent concepts suggest that neutrophils could contribute to periodontitis not only by initiating the lesion but also by participating in its progression, by recruiting T-helper 17 cells or promoting the accumulation of B cells and plasma cells in the established and advanced lesions.

Macrophages are an important source of proinflammatory and potentially destructive molecules for tissues, such as interleukin-1 (IL-1), tumor necrosis factor alpha (TNF-α), MMP, and prostaglandin E_2 [30], which play an important role and are elevated in the gingival tissue and in the gingival crevicular fluid of patients with chronic periodontitis [28]. Therefore, studies have shown a direct correlation of macrophage infiltration with the severity of periodontal disease [31], contributing greatly to the intensification of the degradation of the collagen matrix in the connective periodontal tissue [32, 33]. These macrophages may undergo a classical (M1) or alternative (M2) activation. M1 macrophages are induced by microbial agents (e.g., LPS) or by Th1 cytokines and show high phagocytic capacity and an increased expression of proinflammatory cytokines, costimulatory, and antimicrobial molecules. In contrast, M2 macrophages are induced by Th2 cytokines and secrete high levels of IL-10 and transforming growth factor beta 1 (TGF-β1). Therefore, they have immunoregulatory properties and promote cell proliferation and tissue regeneration [29, 34]. In periodontal inflammation models, macrophages share properties of both M1 and M2. However, M1 macrophages show a predominance over M2 macrophages, suggesting that M1 macrophages probably represent a subset associated with periodontitis [35–37].

3.2.2 Adaptive immune response in periodontal disease

When the inflammatory response becomes chronic, the lymphocytes of the adaptive immune system invade the periodontal tissues releasing inflammatory and immune molecular mediators, which alter the balance of bone metabolism, marking the transition from gingivitis to periodontitis [29]. The activation of lymphocytes requires two types of signals: a signal induced by the antigen receptor itself when recognizing its related antigen and a costimulatory signal by professional antigen-presenting cells (APCs) [22]. In gingivitis, the predominant APCs are CD14[+] and CD83[+] dendritic cells. While in the periodontitis, the predominant APCs are CD19[+] and CD83[+] B lymphocytes [38]. Therefore, the activation of adaptive immunity has a great influence on the bone loss in periodontitis, associated with B and T lymphocytes, since several studies have shown that these cells are the main cellular sources of activator of the κB ligand receptor of the nuclear factor (RANKL) during periodontal inflammation [39].

RANKL is a cytokine member of the TNF family that can be bound or secreted to the membrane and stimulates the differentiation of osteoclasts, cell fusion, and activation that leads to bone resorption [40, 41]. Osteoblasts and stromal cells of the bone marrow predominantly express RANKL bound to the membrane, which induces osteoclastogenesis through cell contact with osteoclast precursors. Likewise, activated T and B cells produce both the membrane-bound and soluble RANKL forms. Soluble RANKL can induce osteoclastogenesis independently of direct contact between infiltrating lymphocytes and osteoclast precursors on the bone surface. However, 17 T-helper cells expressing RANKL, but not T-helper 1 cells, activate osteoclasts also by direct cell-cell contact [42]. In the alveolar bone, the RANKL/OPG/RANK system controls the balance of the bone metabolism [43]. RANKL is the osteoclasts activator and the molecular signal directly responsible for the bone resorption, which interacts with its associated receptor RANK on the surface of osteoclast and osteoclast precursors, which triggers its recruitment on the bone surface and cell fusion and activation [44]. Osteoprotegerin (OPG) is a soluble protein that has the ability to block the biological functions of RANKL by competitive inhibition [45]. In periodontitis, the increase in RANKL/OPG promotes the recruitment of osteoclast precursors, their fusion, and subsequent activation, leading to bone resorption [46].

On the other hand, Th1 lymphocytes have a fundamental role in the establishment and progression of periodontitis, through the increase of IFN-γ levels [18]. Studies have shown that mice IFN-γ-deficient showed low levels of inflammatory cytokines and chemokines, as well as macrophages infiltrated in periodontal tissue, developing a less severe phenotype of alveolar bone destruction [47]. IL-1β and TNF-α are cytokines secreted by Th1 lymphocytes. TNF-α and IL-1β produce vasodilation, stimulate the activation of endothelial cells to increase the recruitment of immune cells, increase the chemokines production in most cell types, participate in the activation of neutrophils, and stimulate secretion and tissue activation of MMPs, among other functions. Although neither IL-1β nor TNF-α is directly involved in the stimulation of bone resorption, they indirectly promote bone destruction by stimulating sustained inflammation of the periodontal tissue [48]. Th2 lymphocytes are the main cellular source of IL-4, which promotes the change of class to the secretion of IgE in B cells and favors the alternative activation of macrophages in an IFN-γ-independent pathway. These effector functions of the Th2 lymphocytes negatively regulate the inflammatory and Th1 lymphocyte responses, so that the polarization of a Th2-type immune response in periodontitis may represent a damaged adaptive immune response [18, 49]. Finally, RANKL can also be secreted by Th17 lymphocytes, which in cooperation with inflammatory cytokines derived from Th1 lymphocytes are capable to tilt bone metabolism favoring bone resorption [50].

4. Conclusion

The main etiological factor of periodontal disease is the bacteria, which are capable of activating the innate immune response of the host inducing an inflammatory response. The evolution of this inflammatory response culminates in the destruction of periodontal tissues. For this reason, it is important to understand the different molecular and cellular mechanisms of the pathogenesis of periodontal disease, with the purpose of making an opportune diagnosis and appropriate treatment and prognosis.

Acknowledgements

Thanks to the authors who collaborated in the writing of this chapter: Dr. en C. José Luis Muñoz-Carrillo, Dra. Viridiana Elizabeth Hernández-Reyes, Dr. Oscar Eduardo García-Huerta, Dra. Karla Mariana Chávez-Ruvalcaba, Dra. en C. Francisca Chávez-Ruvalcaba, Dra. en C. María Isabel Chávez-Ruvalcaba, and Dra. Lizbeth Díaz-Alfaro, as well as the Universities involved, Cuauhtémoc University Aguascalientes, Autonomous University of Zacatecas, and Autonomous University of Aguascalientes for financial support for chapter publication.

Conflict of interest

We have no conflict of interest related to this work.

Author details

José Luis Muñoz-Carrillo[1]*, Viridiana Elizabeth Hernández-Reyes[1], Oscar Eduardo García-Huerta[1], Francisca Chávez-Ruvalcaba[2], María Isabel Chávez-Ruvalcaba[3], Karla Mariana Chávez-Ruvalcaba[4] and Lizbeth Díaz-Alfaro[5]

1 Faculty of Odontology, School of Biomedical Sciences, Cuauhtémoc University Aguascalientes, Aguascalientes, Mexico

2 Nutrition Degree, Health Sciences Area, Autonomous University of Zacatecas, Zacatecas, Mexico

3 Laboratory of Immunoparasitology, Academic Unit of Biological Sciences, Autonomous University of Zacatecas, Zacatecas, Mexico

4 Academic Unit of Odontology, Autonomous University of Zacatecas, Guadalupe, Zacatecas, Mexico

5 Department of Stomatology, Autonomous University of Aguascalientes, Aguascalientes, Mexico

*Address all correspondence to: mcbjlmc@gmail.com

IntechOpen

References

[1] Papapanou PN, Sanz M, Buduneli N, Dietrich T, Feres M, Fine DH, et al. Periodontitis: Consensus report of workgroup 2 of the 2017 world workshop on the classification of periodontal and peri-implant diseases and conditions. Journal of Periodontology. 2018;**89**(Suppl. 1): S173-S182. DOI: 10.1002/JPER.17-0721

[2] Kassebaum NJ, Bernabe E, Dahiya M, Bhandari B, Murray CJ, Marcenes W. Global burden of severe periodontitis in 1990-2010: A systematic review and meta-regression. Journal of Dental Research. 2014;**93**(11):1045-1053

[3] Ansari G, Golpayegani MV, Welbury R. Histology and embryology of the teeth and periodontium. In: Ansari G, Golpayegani MV, Welbury R, editors. Atlas of Pediatric Oral and Dental Developmental Anomalies. Chichester: Wiley; 2018. pp. 13-16. DOI: 10.1002/9781119380894.ch2

[4] Nanci A, Bosshardt DD. Structure of periodontal tissues in health and disease. Periodontology 2000. 2006;**40**(1):11-28. DOI: 10.1111/j.1600-0757.2005.00141.x

[5] Ramos MJ. Biomecánica de los tejidos periodontales. Kiru. 2013;**10**(1):75-82

[6] Lindhe J, Lang NP. Periodontología clínica e implantología odontológica. 6a Edición ed. Madrid, España: Editorial Medica Panamericana S. A de C.V; 2017. pp. 3-37

[7] Hassell TM. Tissues and cells of the periodontium. Periodontology 2000. 1993;**3**(1):9-38. DOI: 10.1111/j.1600-0757.1993.tb00230.x

[8] Cho MI, Garant PR. Development and general structure of the periodontium. Periodontology 2000. 2000;**24**(1):9-27. DOI: 10.1034/j.1600-0757.2000.2240102.x

[9] Pisoschi C, Stanciulescu C, Banita M. Growth factors and connective tissue homeostasis in periodontal disease. In: Buduneli N, editor. Pathogenesis and Treatment of Periodontitis. London: InTechOpen; 2012. pp. 55-80. DOI: 10.5772/33669

[10] Tonetti MS, Greenwell H, Kornman KS. Staging and grading of periodontitis: Framework and proposal of a new classification and case definition. Journal of Periodontology. 2018;**89**(Suppl. 1):S159-S172. DOI: 10.1002/JPER.18-0006

[11] Page RC, Schroeder HE. Pathogenesis of inflammatory periodontal disease. A summary of current work. Laboratory Investigation. 1976;**34**(3):235-249

[12] Kinane DF. Causation and pathogenesis of periodontal disease. Periodontology 2000. 2001;**25**(1):8-20. DOI: 10.1034/j.1600-0757.2001.22250102.x

[13] Bostanci N, Belibasakis GN. Periodontal pathogenesis: Definitions and historical perspectives. In: Bostanci N, Belibasakis G, editors. Pathogenesis of Periodontal Diseases. Cham: Springer; 2018. pp. 1-7. DOI: 10.1007/978-3-319-53737-5_1

[14] Cavalla F, Araujo-Pires AC, Biguetti CC, Garlet GP. Cytokine networks regulating inflammation and immune defense in the oral cavity. Current Oral Health Reports. 2014;**1**(2):104-113. DOI: 10.1007/s40496-014-0016-9

[15] Kornman KS, Page RC, Tonetti MS. The host response to the microbial challenge in periodontitis: Assembling the players. Periodontology 2000. 1997;**14**(1):33-53. DOI: 10.1111/j.1600-0757.1997.tb00191.x

[16] Mira A, Simon-Soro A, Curtis MA. Role of microbial communities in the pathogenesis of periodontal

diseases and caries. Journal of Clinical Periodontology. 2017;**44**(Suppl. 18): S23-S38. DOI: 10.1111/jcpe.12671

[17] Silva N, Abusleme L, Bravo D, Dutzan N, Garcia-Sesnich J, Vernal R, et al. Host response mechanisms in periodontal diseases. Journal of Applied Oral Science. 2015;**23**(3):329-355. DOI: 10.1590/1678-775720140259

[18] Cavalla F, Biguetti CC, Garlet TP, Trombone APF, Garlet GP. Inflammatory pathways of bone resorption in periodontitis. In: Bostanci N, Belibasakis G, editors. Pathogenesis of Periodontal Diseases. Cham: Springer; 2018. pp. 59-85. DOI: 10.1007/978-3-319-53737-5_6

[19] Muñoz Carrillo JL, Castro García FP, Gutiérrez Coronado O, Moreno García MA, Contreras Cordero JF. Physiology and pathology of innate immune response against pathogens. In: Rezaei N, editor. Physiology and Pathology of Immunology. London: InTechOpen; 2017. pp. 99-134. DOI: 10.5772/intechopen.70556

[20] Muñoz-Carrillo JL, Ortega-Martín Del Campo J, Gutiérrez-Coronado O, Villalobos-Gutiérrez PT, Contreras-Cordero JF, Ventura-Juárez J. Adipose tissue and inflammation. In: Szablewski L, editor. Adipose Tissue. London: InTechOpen; 2018. pp. 93-121. DOI: 10.5772/intechopen.74227

[21] Muñoz-Carrillo JL, Contreras-Cordero JF, Gutiérrez-Coronado O, Villalobos-Gutiérrez PT, Ramos-Gracia LG, Hernández-Reyes VE. Cytokine Profiling Plays a Crucial Role in Activating Immune System to Clear Infectious Pathogens. London: IntechOpen. DOI: 10.5772/intechopen.80843

[22] Muñoz-Carrillo JL, Castro-García FP, Chávez-Rubalcaba F, Chávez-Rubalcaba I, Martínez-Rodríguez JL, Hernández-Ruiz ME. Immune system disorders: Hypersensitivity and autoimmunity. In: Athari SS, editor. Immunoregulatory Aspects of Immunotherapy. London: InTechOpen. pp. 1-30. DOI: 10.5772/intechopen.75794

[23] Noguchi S, Ukai T, Kuramoto A, Yoshinaga Y, Nakamura H, Takamori Y, et al. The histopathological comparison on the destruction of the periodontal tissue between normal junctional epithelium and long junctional epithelium. Journal of Periodontal Research. 2017;**52**(1):74-82. DOI: 10.1111/jre.12370

[24] Cavalla F, Osorio C, Paredes R, Valenzuela MA, García-Sesnich J, Sorsa T, et al. Matrix metalloproteinases regulate extracellular levels of SDF-1/CXCL12, IL-6 and VEGF in hydrogen peroxide-stimulated human periodontal ligament fibroblasts. Cytokine. 2015;**73**(1):114-121. DOI: 10.1016/j.cyto.2015.02.001

[25] Han MX, Ding C, Kyung HM. Genetic polymorphisms in pattern recognition receptors and risk of periodontitis: Evidence based on 12,793 subjects. Human Immunology. 2015;**76**(7):496-504. DOI: 10.1016/j.humimm.2015.06.006

[26] Song B, Zhang YL, Chen LJ, Zhou T, Huang WK, Zhou X, et al. The role of Toll-like receptors in periodontitis. Oral Diseases. 2017;**23**(2):168-180. DOI: 10.1111/odi.12468

[27] Pöllänen MT, Laine MA, Ihalin R, Uitto VJ. Host-bacteria crosstalk at the dentogingival junction. International Journal of Dentistry. 2012;**2012**(821383):1-14. DOI: 10.1155/2012/821383

[28] Kang W, Hu Z, Ge S. Healthy and inflamed gingival fibroblasts differ in their inflammatory response to Porphyromlonas gingivalis lipopolysaccharide. Inflammation.

2016;**39**(5):1842-1852. DOI: 10.1007/
s10753-016-0421-4

[29] Hajishengallis G, Korostoff JM.
Revisiting the Page & Schroeder model:
The good, the bad and the unknowns
in the periodontal host response 40
years later. Periodontology 2000.
2017;**75**(1):116-151. DOI: 10.1111/
prd.12181

[30] Cekici A, Kantarci A, Hasturk
H, Van Dyke TE. Inflammatory and
immune pathways in the pathogenesis
of periodontal disease. Periodontology
2000. 2014;**64**(1):57-80. DOI: 10.1111/
prd.12002

[31] Gupta M, Chaturvedi R, Jain A. Role
of monocyte chemoattractant protein-1
(MCP-1) as an immune-diagnostic
biomarker in the pathogenesis of
chronic periodontal disease. Cytokine.
2013;**61**(3):892-897. DOI: 10.1016/j.
cyto.2012.12.012

[32] Bodet C, Chandad F, Grenier D.
Inflammatory responses of a
macrophage/epithelial cell co-culture
model to mono and mixed infections
with *Porphyromonas gingivalis*,
Treponema denticola, and *Tannerella
forsythia*. Microbes and Infection.
2006;**8**(1):27-35. DOI: 10.1016/j.
micinf.2005.05.015

[33] Kiili M, Cox SW, Chen HY,
Wahlgren J, Maisi P, Eley BM,
et al. Collagenase-2 (MMP-8) and
collagenase-3 (MMP-13) in adult
periodontitis: Molecular forms and
levels in gingival crevicular fluid and
immunolocalisation in gingival tissue.
Journal of Clinical Periodontology.
2002;**29**(3):224-232. DOI:
10.1034/j.1600-051x.2002.290308.x

[34] Braga TT, Agudelo JS, Camara NO.
Macrophages during the fibrotic
process: M2 as friend and foe. Frontiers
in Immunology. 2015;**6**:602. DOI:
10.3389/fimmu.2015.00602

[35] Gonzalez OA, Novak MJ, Kirakodu
S, Stromberg A, Nagarajan R, Huang
CB, et al. Differential gene expression
profiles reflecting macrophage
polarization in aging and periodontitis
gingival tissues. Immunological
Investigations. 2015;**44**(7):643-664.
DOI: 10.3109/08820139.2015.107026

[36] Yu T, Zhao L, Huang X, Ma C, Wang
Y, Zhang J, et al. Enhanced activity of
the macrophage M1/M2 phenotypes and
phenotypic switch to M1 in periodontal
infection. Journal of Periodontology.
2016;**87**(9):1092-1102. DOI: 10.1902/
jop.2016.160081

[37] Lam RS, O'Brien-Simpson NM,
Lenzo JC, Holden JA, Brammar GC,
Walsh KA, et al. Macrophage depletion
abates *Porphyromonas gingivalis*-induced
alveolar bone resorption in mice. Journal
of Immunology. 2014;**193**(5):2349-2362.
DOI: 10.4049/jimmunol.1400853

[38] Gemmell E, Seymour GJ. Cytokine
profiles of cells extracted from humans
with periodontal diseases. Journal of
Dental Research. 1998;**77**(1):16-26. DOI:
10.1177/00220345980770010101

[39] Dutzan N, Gamonal J, Silva A,
Sanz M, Vernal R. Over-expression of
forkhead box P3 and its association
with receptor activator of nuclear
factor-kappa B ligand, interleukin
(IL)-17, IL-10 and transforming
growth factor-beta during the
progression of chronic periodontitis.
Journal of Clinical Periodontology.
2009;**36**(5):396-403. DOI:
10.1111/j.1600-051X.2009.01390.x

[40] Nakashima T, Hayashi M,
Takayanagi H. New insights into
osteoclastogenic signaling mechanisms.
Trends in Endocrinology and
Metabolism. 2012;**23**(11):582-590. DOI:
10.1016/j.tem.2012.05.005

[41] Kim JH, Kim N. Regulation of
NFATc1 in osteoclast differentiation.
Journal of Bone Metabolism.

2014;**21**(4):233-241. DOI: 10.11005/jbm.2014.21.4.233

[42] Kikuta J, Wada Y, Kowada T, Wang Z, Sun-Wada GH, Nishiyama I, et al. Dynamic visualization of RANKL and Th17-mediated osteoclast function. The Journal of Clinical Investigation. 2013;**123**(2):866-873. DOI: 10.1172/JCI65054

[43] Belibasakis GN, Bostanci N. The RANKL-OPG system in clinical periodontology. Journal of Clinical Periodontology. 2012;**39**(3):239-248. DOI: 10.1111/j.1600-051X.2011.01810.x

[44] Lee JW, Kobayashi Y, Nakamichi Y, Udagawa N, Takahashi N, Im NK, et al. Alisol-B, a novel phyto-steroid, suppresses the RANKL-induced osteoclast formation and prevents bone loss in mice. Biochemical Pharmacology. 2010;**80**(3):352-361. DOI: 10.1016/j.bcp.2010.04.014

[45] Hofbauer LC, Neubauer A, Heufelder AE. Receptor activator of nuclear factor-kappaB ligand and osteoprotegerin: Potential implications for the pathogenesis and treatment of malignant bone diseases. Cancer. 2001;**92**(3):460-470. DOI: 10.1002/1097-0142(20010801)92:3<460::AID-CNCR1344>3.0.CO;2-D

[46] Menezes R, Garlet TP, Letra A, Bramante CM, Campanelli AP, Figueira Rde C, et al. Differential patterns of receptor activator of nuclear factor kappa B ligand/osteoprotegerin expression in human periapical granulomas: Possible association with progressive or stable nature of the lesions. Journal of Endodontia. 2008;**34**(8):932-938. DOI: 10.1016/j.joen.2008.05.002

[47] Garlet GP, Cardoso CR, Campanelli AP, Garlet TP, Avila-Campos MJ, Cunha FQ, et al. The essential role of IFN-gamma in the control of lethal *Aggregatibacter actinomycetemcomitans* infection in mice. Microbes and Infection. 2008;**10**(5):489-496. DOI: 10.1016/j.micinf.2008.01.010

[48] Preshaw PM, Taylor JJ. How has research into cytokine interactions and their role in driving immune responses impacted our understanding of periodontitis? Journal of Clinical Periodontology. 2011;**38**(Suppl. 11):60-84. DOI: 10.1111/j.1600-051X.2010.01671.x

[49] Gemmell E, Yamazaki K, Seymour GJ. The role of T cells in periodontal disease: Homeostasis and autoimmunity. Periodontology 2000. 2007;**43**:14-40. DOI: 10.1111/j.1600-0757.2006.00173.x

[50] Cardoso CR, Garlet GP, Crippa GE, Rosa AL, Júnior WM, Rossi MA, et al. Evidence of the presence of T helper type 17 cells in chronic lesions of human periodontal disease. Oral Microbiology and Immunology. 2009;**24**(1):1-6. DOI: 10.1111/j.1399-302X.2008.00463.x

Section 2

How to Diagnose
Periodontal Diseases

Chapter 2

Use of Biomarkers for the Diagnosis of Periodontitis

Javier González-Ramírez, Nicolás Serafín-Higuera,
Marina Concepción Silva Mancilla,
Gustavo Martínez-Coronilla, Jesús Famanía-Bustamante
and Ana Laura López López

Abstract

Periodontal disease is the most common oral condition of human population; if periodontitis is not treated in its initial stages, it can cause the loss of teeth. The diagnosis of periodontitis is based on clinical measurements. However, currently with the advancement of technology, other diagnostic and monitoring options are being search. In fact, different types of biomarkers have been evaluated where different biological fluids have been used as a source of the sample. We will try to summarize existing biomarkers of different periodontitis stages and make a comparison of the periodontal biomarkers evaluated so far and their usefulness in diagnosis and monitoring of periodontitis.

Keywords: biomarkers, periodontitis, dentobacterial plaque, gingivitis

1. Introduction

Health in general is fundamental in humans, oral health plays an important role, and any alteration in it can influence the general welfare of individuals. Diseases of the oral cavity are very important due to its high incidence and prevalence according to the World Health Organization [1].

Regarding the epidemiology of the disease, we can say that from 5 to 15% of the population of the United States suffers from severe periodontitis [2]. Data from the Department of Health of Mexico mention that approximately 8.8% of the Mexican population has chronic periodontitis. This is more common among subjects 35 years of age and older, where it is estimated that the frequency is 22% [3].

Periodontitis is a chronic inflammatory disease that compromises the integrity of the tissues that support the teeth, which include the gingiva, periodontal ligament, dental cement, and alveolar bone, and are collectively known as the periodontium [4, 5].

This disease is caused by specific microorganisms or groups of specific microorganisms, which in the end produce a greater formation of probing depth, recession, or both. When these conditions remain, they cause the tissue to be destroyed and the tooth to be lost. This disturbs the mastication, phonation, and esthetics of the patient, which affect the quality of life [4].

The traditional treatment for periodontitis decreases the microbial presence by means of the mechanical interruption and the elimination of the bacterial layers that form in the surfaces of the teeth and adjacent soft tissues [2].

In the pathology of periodontitis, the clinical, radiographic, and histological characteristics of the gingival groove and pouch epithelium, the underlying connective tissue and the types of resident and infiltrating blood cells in the initial, early, established periodontal injury are known [6].

Currently, the diagnosis requires rapidity, sensitivity, and specificity since determining the stage in which the patient is located is fundamental for a good treatment; for this reason molecules are currently being sought that vary when the person is healthy and when the person has the disease. However, despite all the researches that exist regarding chronic inflammation, the diagnosis of periodontitis is based on clinical measurements; these not only show low sensitivity and specificity as diagnostic tests but are also subjective and laborious. The objective of this chapter is to try to describe what a biomarker is, the types of biomarkers evaluated in periodontitis, the sources to obtain these biomarkers, and their usefulness.

2. Biomarkers

The definition of biomarkers as established by the National Institute of Health (NIH) is as follows: biomarkers are the biological, biochemical, anthropometric, physiological, etc. characteristics, which are objectively measurable, capable of identifying physiological or pathological processes, or a pharmacological response or a therapeutic intervention [7].

There are different types of biomarkers; the ideal biomarker must be specific, sensitive, predictive, rapid, economical, noninvasive, and stable in vivo and in vitro. Additionally, it must have enough preclinical and clinical relevance to modify decisions regarding the pathological process in which applies [7].

Before a biological marker is used in human health studies, its validation is fundamental; therefore, the selection and approval process requires careful consideration of specificity and sensitivity, establishing accuracy, precision, quality assurance, analytical procedure, and interpretation of measurement data, which must be compared with other variables [8].

3. Biomarkers for the diagnosis of periodontitis

3.1 Importance of the different biomarkers used for the diagnosis of periodontitis

Because there are certain molecules, like trace elements, proteins (cytokines), and proteolytic enzymes, these have been considered as possible biomarkers of periodontal disease, we will try to discuss the relevance of these groups below.

3.1.1 Proteins (cytokines) involved in the inflammatory process of periodontitis

Inflammation has evolved as a protective response to an injury, is a primordial response that eliminates or neutralizes foreign organisms or materials, in general; the innate inflammatory response starts in minutes and, if all is well, resolves in a matter of hours. In contrast, chronic inflammation persists for weeks, months, or even years [9]. The inflammatory response that occurs in periodontal disease is mediated mainly by B and T lymphocytes, neutrophils, and monocytes/macrophages. These are activated to produce inflammatory mediators, including cytokines and chemokines [10]. Several pro-inflammatory cytokines including interleukins like IL-1, IL-6, IL-12, IL-17, IL-18, and IL-21; tumor necrosis factor alpha (TNFα); and interferon (IFN-γ) have been demonstrated to be involved in the pathogenesis of periodontitis [2].

3.1.2 Metalloproteinases

There is significant evidence showing that collagenases, along with other matrix metalloproteinases, play an important role in periodontal tissue destruction. The main group of enzymes responsible for the collagen and other protein degradation in extracellular matrix (ECM) is matrix metalloproteinases (MMPs) [11]. Several works have shown that matrix metalloproteinases are upregulated in periodontal inflammation; transcription of matrix metalloproteinase genes is very low in healthy periodontal tissue. In periodontal disease, secretion of specific matrix metalloproteinases is stimulated or downregulated by various cytokines [12].

3.1.3 Calcium

The importance of calcium in the development of periodontal disease has been recognized since the 1980s [13]. In addition to this, a relationship has been found between people who suffer from periodontitis and who also have osteoporosis [14].

3.1.4 Alkaline phosphate

Alkaline phosphatase (ALP) is an intracellular enzyme. It is considered that when this enzyme increases in saliva, it can be determined that there is inflammation and destruction of healthy tissues [15]. It is worth mentioning that other enzymes representative of tissue degradation are aspartate aminotransferase (AST), alanine aminotransferase (ALT), gamma-glutamyl transferase (GGT), alkaline phosphatase (ALP), and acid phosphatase (ACP) [16].

3.1.5 Phosphate

Phosphorus is an essential element and plays an important role in multiple biological processes, due to the fact that maintaining physiological phosphate balance is of crucial biological importance for bone health [17]. Approximately 85% of phosphorus is in the bone, primarily compounded with calcium (Ca^{2+}), the most abundant mineral in hydroxyapatite (HAP) crystals deposited on the collagen matrix [18].

The importance of phosphate in periodontal disease has been observed in X-linked hypophosphatemia (XLH); this disease is a rare skeletal genetic illness in which increased phosphate in the kidney produces hypophosphatemia and prevents normal mineralization of the bone and bone dentine. In a study of 2017, it was observed that the frequency and severity of periodontitis increased in adults with XLH and that the severity varied according to the treatment of hypophosphatemia. Patients who benefited from early and continuous phosphate supplementation during childhood had less loss of periodontal attachment than patients with late or incomplete supplementation [19].

3.1.6 pH

Although the pH of the oral cavity is between 5 and 9, it is also known to vary widely depending on several factors. There are studies that report that there is a statistically significant correlation between pH and periodontal pocket formation [20].

3.1.7 Oxidative stress

Periodontitis is an inflammatory disease of the supporting tissues of the teeth, it is defined as a complex infectious disease that results from the interaction of the bacterial infection and the response of the host to the bacterial challenge, and the disease is modified by environmental factors, acquired risk factors, and genetic susceptibility [21]. In recent years, the inflammatory response has been associated with oxidative stress, specifically with reactive oxygen species since it is considered to play a central role in the progression of many inflammatory diseases [22].

Oxidative stress create multiple products in affected tissues, such as reactive oxygen species which are free radicals and other non-radical derivatives which are involved in normal cell metabolism [23], other metabolites can damage DNA such as 8-hydroxy2'-deoxyguanosine (8-OHdG) or 8-oxo-7,8-dihydro-2'-deoxyguanosine (8-oxodG) which are two of the predominant forms of free radicals induced by oxidative lesions. In fact, 8-oxodG has been widely used as a biomarker for oxidative stress [24].

3.1.8 Telopeptide

Bone resorption is a basic physiological process that is central to the under-standing of many key pathologies, with its most common oral manifestation seen as the alveolar bone destruction in periodontitis [25]. The osteoid matrix consists principally of collagen (90%), other smaller proteins, and proteoglycans. The main structural protein of the bone is type I collagen. Consequently, most available bone resorption markers are based on degradation products of type I collagen. According to Koizumi et al. [26], ICTP (telopeptide) is one of the best markers for clinical use.

3.1.9 miRNAs (microRNAs)

Nowadays, RNAs that do not code for protein have taken on great importance because, in addition to maintaining their importance in the determination of cellular phenotypes [27], now they are recognized as dynamic participants in the performance of cellular activities [28].

It has been mentioned and demonstrated that miRNAs are involved in bone metabolism, in fact, some studies have shown that they are associated with the activa-tor of the nuclear factor receptor kappa-B ligand (RANKL) induced osteoclastogen-esis. Within these miRNAs, miR-223 [29] was the first to associate with periodontal tissue, although other miRNAs such as miR-15a, miR-29b, miR-125a, miR-146a, miR148 / 148a, miR-223 and miR-92 have been identified more recently as important in periodontal health and have even been considered potential biomarkers [30].

3.1.10 Other markers of periodontal disease

Other biomarkers have been analyzed to determine periodontitis. One of these is chondroitin sulfate, which is a natural glycosaminoglycan (GAG) present in the extracellular matrix [31]; chondroitin sulfate is recognized for its immunomodula-tory effects, such as the reduction of nuclear translocation NF-κB, the decrease in the production of pro-inflammatory cytokines interleukin-1β (IL-1β) and tumor necrosis factor alpha (TNF-α), and the decrease in expression and activity of nitric oxide synthase-2 (NOS-2) and cyclooxygenase-2 (COX-2) [32]. Another molecule that has been proposed as a possible biomarker is MUC-4. Mucins are high-molecular-weight glycoproteins, are involved in diverse biological functions, are members of trans-membrane mucin family, and are expressed in airway epithelial cells and body fluids like saliva, tear film, ear fluid, and breast milk [33]. It has been reported that the production of MUC-4 could be regulated by inflammatory cytokines [34].

3.2 Biomarkers determined in saliva

Saliva is a seromucous secretion, consisting of 99% water; however, saliva is also composed of glycoproteins, phosphate ions, bicarbonate, sodium, chlorine, fluorine, calcium, and potassium and has a neutral pH [35], which forms a film of liquid consistency that covers the surface of the oral mucosa, with the purpose of lubricating it and keeping it moist among many other characteristics for the maintenance of oral health [36]. The composition of saliva varies from one place to another in the oral cavity of each individual [35]. If there are changes in its composition, there may be significant alterations in deterioration of the health of the host [37].

Due to the described characteristics of saliva, several authors have claimed that these salivary constituents may actually be useful indicators of both local and systemic disorders. These revelations have formed the basis of the field of saliva diagnosis and, therefore, have triggered research that culminated in the identification of saliva-based biomarkers for disorders ranging from cancer to infectious diseases [38]. In addition to the above, saliva has several advantages when compared to other sources for diagnosing diseases since saliva is easily collected and stored and ideal for early detection of disease as it contains specific soluble biological markers [39]. Saliva has been used to diagnose diseases as diverse as autoimmune disorders, cardiovascular diseases, diabetes, HIV, oral cancer, and oral diseases [40].

3.2.1 Proteins (cytokines) determined in saliva that could be used as biomarkers

In our review we observed that there are about 15 works that were dedicated to investigate the possible use of these proteins determined in saliva as biomarkers to determine periodontitis. We can say that of all the works, the majority focuses on comparing healthy groups with periodontitis; only three researches include the group of gingivitis, which indicates that this group should be used more for this type of studies. We need to remember that gingivitis is considered an intermediate stage that may or may not lead to periodontitis [41], and if the patient performs good dental hygiene in combination with the treatment, in general, progression to periodontitis can also be stopped [42].

On the other hand, the cytokine that has been most explored and that better results have given as biomarkers to detect in saliva is the cytokine IL-1β [43–48]; this must be due to the recognized importance of interleukin-1β, as an important mediator in the pathophysiology of periodontitis [49].

However, other cytokines such as IL-6 and IL-2 have also been explored [43, 44, 48, 50]; IL-6 is recognized for playing a role as a pro-inflammatory cytokine acting on bone resorption in the presence of infections [51]. Regarding IL-2, a study that investigated cytokine profiles at different stages of the development of periodontitis found that levels of mRNA for IL-2 were significantly associated with the phase of resolution of the disease [52]. This agrees with reports that IL-2 has been implicated in the stimulation of osteoclasts [53].

Regarding MCP-1, Gupta et al. [54] conducted a study in 45 patients with an average age of 43 years for healthy patients and 41 for patients with periodontitis, with results similar to Nisha et al. [55]. In both studies it was found that the levels of MCP-1 in saliva can be a good biomarker for the development of periodontal disease. One difference between the studies is that Nisha's work included a group of patients with gingivitis, while Gupta's study does not include it.

Regarding the possibility of using prostaglandin E2 (PGE2) as biomarkers in saliva to diagnose gingivitis, Syndergaard et al. [56] conducted a study with 80 participants, 40 without gingivitis and 40 with gingivitis, and found that the levels of PGE2 in the group with gingivitis were significantly higher compared with the control group. This study reported that PGE2 remained high after prophylaxis. As for other studies conducted with the purpose of comparing the concentrations of PGE2, Sanchez et al. [82] conducted a study in which the population was 74 adult subjects who were grouped according to the progress of the periodontal disease in mild, moderate, and severe; the conclusion was that the levels of PGE2 increase as the severity of the periodontal disease progressed. In addition a high sensitivity and specificity were reported.

When TNF-α is evaluated as a possible biomarker for the diagnosis of periodontitis, we found that there are discrepancies since in some studies, such as Eivazi et al. [57] who conducted a study with one healthy group and another with chronic periodontitis which reported that before and after starting treatment, the concentrations of TNF-α in saliva were higher in the healthy group than in the periodontitis group. In contrary to the results reported by Yue et al. [48], they found that TNF-α concentrations were higher in the saliva of patients with advanced periodontitis than in the saliva of healthy subjects. Yue's study is supported by studies that investigate the loss of the alveolar bone since the concentration of TNF-α in subjects with alveolar resorption is low [58].

Yue et al. [48] found that in the saliva of patients with aggressive periodontitis (AP) have higher levels of IFN-γ in the saliva compared to subjects without AP; this decrease was statistically significant throughout the course of treatment (p < 0.05).

3.2.2 Metalloproteinases

Matrix metalloproteinases (MMPs) are key proteases involved in destructive periodontal diseases. A total of 23 MMPs have been described. These MMPs can be found in periodontal tissues as pro-forms, active forms, complex species, fragmented, and cell-bound species [59]. MMPs are the most important group of proteinases responsible for the degradation of extracellular matrix proteins during periodontitis, and any imbalance between MMPs and their inhibitors can trigger the degradation of the ECM, the basement membrane, and the alveolar bone [60].

In this way and due to the importance of MMPs, several researchers have been dedicated to try to determine if MMPs are opportune as biomarkers. Gursoy et al. [61] did a study with the objective of detecting possible markers of periodontitis in saliva, with high sensitivity and specificity; to determine this, the salivary concentrations of MMP-8, MMP-9, and MMP-13 among others were measured in 230 subjects. The concentrations of MMP-8, MMP-9, and MMP-13 in saliva were higher in subjects with generalized periodontitis than in controls; however, according to the authors, MMP-8 was the only marker capable of differentiating subjects with severe bone loss of those who presented mild bone loss, so they consider that MMP-8 is a strong candidate to detect alveolar bone destruction [61]. These results were corroborated by Rathnayake et al. [46] who found that MMP-8 could be used as a marker of periodontal disease in large patient populations. An interesting fact that they reported is that smokers compared to non-smokers showed slightly lower concentrations of MMP-8.

Another interesting fact regarding MMP-8 by Ebersole et al. [25] in a study that included 30 healthy volunteers and 50 patients diagnosed with chronic periodontitis is that MMP-8 (among others) was investigated as a biomarker associated with inflammatory and destructive processes of periodontal disease and reported that the levels of MMP-8 of patients who have periodontitis are very different from the normal levels found in healthy subjects and showed a particular diagnostic potential.

Morelli et al. [50] examined 168 participants and found higher salivary levels of matrix metalloproteinases, MMP-3, MMP-8, and MMP-9, in diseased groups compared to healthy. In the same year, Miricescu et al. [62] carried out a study where 20 patients were also included with chronic periodontitis and 20 controls and different biomarkers were evaluated including matrix MMP-8, and as a result it was found that the levels of MMP-8 were significantly increased in patients with chronic periodontitis compared to controls.

Ebersole et al. [43] conducted a study that included 65 healthy subjects, 43 subjects with gingivitis, and 101 subjects with periodontitis. In this study, the levels of MMP-8 very similar to the previous studies stood out in a significant way in the group of periodontitis compared to those of gingivitis and healthy subjects. In a more categorical way, Borujeni et al. [63] reported that MMP-8 provides a substantial sensitivity with which physicians can use the test for MMP-8 and thus detect periodontitis in their patients.

Similarly, Gupta et al. [64] made an investigation with the objective of establishing MMP-8 as a noninvasive marker for the early diagnosis of chronic periodontitis. The study included 40 subjects who were divided into two groups: 20 healthy subjects and 20 patients with chronic periodontitis. The results of this study demonstrate high concentrations of MMP-8 in individuals with chronic periodontitis.

Already Lira et al. [65] continued to explore the importance of MMP-8 and conducted a study that aimed to evaluate the levels of markers related to innate immunity, the MMP-8 in the saliva from patients with aggressive generalized periodontitis, and patients with gingivitis and healthy. In the saliva, MMP-8 levels were higher in aggressive periodontitis than in healthy patients; in this way it is reaffirmed that MMP-8 can be an important biomarker of periodontitis.

Other researchers such as Virtanen et al. [66] continued to look for other metalloproteinases as potential biomarkers, and some reaffirm that the salivary concentrations of matrix metalloproteinases such as MMP-8 and MMP-9 are slightly higher in patients with periodontitis, although they report that the differences between the groups were not significant. Interestingly, this group reports that MMP-13 values were significantly higher in the group without periodontitis compared to patients with periodontitis and also report that the concentration of MMP-13 may have some gender implications in periodontitis.

Following with the MMP-8, Mauramo et al. [67] studied whether the levels of MMP-8 in the saliva are associated with periodontitis in 258 subjects. Periodontitis was more frequent among subjects with high levels of MMP-8 in the saliva. The highest levels of salivary MMP-8 were associated with any periodontal diagnosis (mild, moderate, or severe). They concluded that elevated levels of MMP-8 in the saliva are associated with periodontitis in a normal adult population.

3.2.3 Calcium

When we search for studies that have explored the detection of calcium present in saliva as a biomarker, we find that while some studies report the usefulness of calcium because the subjects in the periodontitis group had significantly higher levels of salivary calcium than gingivitis and healthy group [68, 69], another work find that high salivary calcium content can be correlated with good dental health but not with periodontal bone destruction [70].

3.2.4 Phosphorus

According to Patel et al. [69] study, phosphorus can be considered a biomarker for the diagnosis of sick and healthy periodontal tissues. The study concludes that as the severity of periodontal disease increases, it also increases total phosphorus levels.

3.2.5 Alkaline phosphatase

Alkaline phosphatase has been evaluated in saliva as a possible biomarker for the detection of periodontitis. Dabra and Singh [16] first study 20 healthy subjects with gingivitis, and 20 with chronic periodontitis were included. This investigation showed a statistically significant increase in alkaline phosphatase activities in the saliva of patients with periodontal disease compared to the control group. A recent study of Patel et al. [69] included 150 healthy subjects, 50 patients with chronic generalized gingivitis, and 50 with periodontitis. In this study it was shown that alkaline phosphatase can be considered for the diagnosis of diseased and healthy periodontal tissues; since as the severity of periodontal disease increases, it also increases alkaline phosphatase levels.

3.2.6 pH

The pH of the saliva has been evaluated, and it has been found that there is a significant change in the pH depending on the severity of the periodontal condition, so the pH can be useful as a rapid diagnostic biomarker in the consultation. The study suggests that the pH becomes alkaline when patients have chronic gingivitis, but it becomes acidic when there is periodontitis [71].

3.2.7 Telopeptide (ICTP)

A 2015 study found that the concentrations of ICTP were higher in the group with periodontitis and lower in the group with healthy patients; this study suggests that the level of ICTP in saliva increases as the patient presents with gingivitis and periodontitis, since the periodontitis samples had the maximum concentration of salivary ICTP. The authors suggest that more studies with a larger sample size be conducted to establish a correlation between the concentrations of ICTP and the individual clinical parameters [72].

3.3 Biomarkers determined in crevicular fluid

In the oral cavity, we find three fluids: the gingival crevicular fluid, the serum, and the total saliva. The gingival crevicular fluid is an exudate, and at present the quantification of its constituents is a current method to identify specific biomarkers with a reasonable sensitivity [73].

The gingival crevicular fluid is an exudate secreted by the gums that can be found in the crevices located at the point where the gumline meets the teeth. The concentrations of this fluid are usually low but may increase when an inflammatory process occurs in the oral cavity [74].

It is considered that due to the noninvasive and simple nature of its collection, the analysis crevicular fluid can be beneficial in determining the periodontal status [75].

3.3.1 Proteins (cytokines) involved in the inflammatory process of periodontitis

Regarding the cytokines that have been evaluated, we can say that they are very similar to those that were evaluated in the saliva; besides that the results are also similar since it has been found that IL-β is the most important cytokine since diverse studies confirm high levels in periodontal disease compared to healthy [48, 76, 77].

In the same way it happens with IL-2 and IL-6, where several studies conclude that both interleukins are important as biomarkers to identify patients with periodontal disease [48, 76, 78].

Regarding MCP-1, the levels of this biomarker were significantly higher in crevicular fluid than healthy subjects ($p < 0.001$) [54].

Regarding IFN-γ and TNF-α, both biomarkers were significantly higher in patients with aggressive periodontitis; this correlates with the findings in saliva where both biomarkers were elevated in sick patients [48].

3.3.2 Metalloproteinases

With respect to metalloproteinases, studies of biomarkers in crevicular fluid have shown that MMP-7 could be useful as a potential new biomarker for periodontitis [79]. Similar to that determined in saliva, MMP-8 is increased in patients with periodontitis and provides a good sensitive measure to establish differences between patients and healthy individuals [77]. It is also useful as a complementary tool in the periodontal diagnosis [67]. Another metalloproteinase that has proved useful is MMP-9. This metalloproteinase correlates with clinical measures and results in good sensitivity to predict the progression of periodontal disease [77].

3.3.3 Alkaline phosphatase

A study was conducted to determine the usefulness of alkaline phosphatase as a biomarker, and this study showed a correlation with the clinical characteristics when mediated in crevicular fluid [80].

3.3.4 miRNAs

According to Mico et al. [81], epigenetic regulation by miRNAs has not yet been studied in periodontal disease using crevicular fluid. They analyzed the possible use as biomarkers of six miRNAs: miR-671, miR-122, miR-1306, miR-27a, miR-223, and miR-1226. Of the six miRNAs analyzed, only miR-1226 can be used as a promising biomarker for periodontal disease since it had statistically significant differences between the healthy group and patients with periodontitis.

3.3.5 Oxidative stress

As previously mentioned, 8-OhdG is a marker of DNA damage and is considered a biomarker to detect oxidative stress [24], that is why it is not surprising that its usefulness as a biomarker of periodontitis was explored. This study was conducted in crevicular fluid, and it could be determined that evaluating this biomarker in crevicular fluid is more effective than in saliva and that it can be useful as a biomarker for determining periodontitis since according to the authors, the severity of the periodontal disease can be revealed [82].

3.3.6 Telopeptide

Telopeptide has also been evaluated as a biomarker in periodontitis in the study by Aruna [83], which suggests that this biomarker could be useful as a specific marker of bone turnover in patients with periodontitis.

3.3.7 Other markers of periodontal disease

Chondroitin sulfate is a biomarker that, due to its results in patients with chronic periodontitis, suggests that it is important in the diagnosis to evaluate the severity of alveolar destruction [80]. MUC4 protein was measured in crevicular fluid and according to this study can be considered as a new biomarker to rule out patients with periodontitis from healthy ones (p < 0.01) [79].

3.3.8 Osteoprotegerin (OPG)

A final marker that we have considered for crevicular fluid is osteoprotegerin; this biomarker was studied by Kinney et al. [77]. They studied healthy patients, with gingivitis and periodontitis, finding that the biomarker OPG was elevated in patients with periodontal disease with a significant difference when compared with healthy patients, so they conclude that this biomarker has a good sensitivity to rule out periodontal disease of gingival health.

3.4 Biomarkers determined in serum

Serum in humans is a matrix commonly used in clinical and biological studies. Many authors recommend using the correct matrix. Both plasma and serum are derived from whole blood that has undergone different biochemical processes after blood extraction. The serum is obtained from the blood that has been clotted [84].

3.4.1 Proteins (cytokines) involved in the inflammatory process of periodontitis

In a study conducted by Nile et al. [85], interleukin IL-17 was identified as a reliable biomarker in 40 patients with chronic periodontitis, later these subjects underwent periodontal therapy, and the values of this interleukin decreased; thus, they consider that IL-17 can be a valuable protein to monitor healing processes after a periodontal intervention.

Another protein related to the immune response MCP-1 was studied by Boström et al. [86]. They studied healthy patients with periodontitis and detected that the MCP-1 protein was increased in the serum and inflamed connective tissue comparing it with healthy patients. In this way, they considered that MCP-1 can help identify patients with periodontitis.

3.4.2 Metalloproteinases

Within the metalloproteinases studied in serum, Lira et al. [65] reported that MMP-8 is elevated in patients with aggressive generalized periodontitis compared with the rest of the patients.

3.4.3 Oxidative stress

Sreeram et al. [87] studied the transpeptidase biomarker (GGT) in healthy subjects and with periodontitis. This biomarker showed elevated levels in patients with periodontitis with respect to healthy. Among the conclusions found in this study was the GGT is useful, economic, and easy to use.

Onder et al [88] studied 4-hydroxynonenal (4-HNE) as a biomarker in serum, concluding that biomarker 4-HNE was at high levels in patients with periodontitis.

In another serum study, other biomarkers of oxidative stress as total antioxidant capacity (TOS) and oxidative stress index (OSI) used in patients with periodontitis and healthy found high levels of TOS and OSI in patients with chronic periodontitis, this suggests that these biomarkers play important roles in periodontitis [89].

3.4.4 Others

Calprotectin was studied by Lira et al. [65]; this biomarker was analyzed in patients with aggressive generalized periodontitis, found elevated levels in these patients compared with healthy and with gingivitis. In addition to the previous study, Nizam et al. [90] studied myeloperoxidase (MOP) and found that it increases in patients with generalized periodontitis compared to healthy ones; nevertheless Meschiari et al. [91] reported similar levels in patients with periodontitis and healthy. This discrepancy between both authors is possible due to the demographic variation and probably the anatomical site where the sample was extracted for analysis.

3.5 Biomarkers determined in plasma

Blood can be a universal reflection of the state or phenotype. Its cellular components are erythrocytes, thrombocytes, and lymphocytes. The liquid portion is called plasma, when all the components are retained. The concentrations of various plasma components are routinely determined in clinical practice [92]. In this way, it is not surprising that biomarkers are sought in plasma.

3.5.1 Proteins (cytokines) involved in the inflammatory process of periodontitis

Among the cytokines evaluated in plasma, we can say that IL-8 and IL-10 were useful to discriminate patients with aggressive periodontitis from healthy ones, and we can add that they were interleukins different from those expressed in the crevicular fluid where IL-2 and IL-6 were relevant [78].

On the other hand, IFN-γ is a biomarker that has been determined in plasma and was significantly high in patients with aggressive periodontitis, this correlates with the findings in crevicular fluid where this biomarker was elevated in sick patients [78].

Regarding MIP-1α, when it was determined in plasma, it was determined that it could be useful to discriminate patients with aggressive periodontitis from healthy ones, since it was found to be elevated [78].

4. Discussion

Periodontitis is one of the most prevalent illnesses in humans [93]. One of the main challenges faced by the periodontics field is to improve the methods for diagnostic and prognostic of periodontitis [94]. Biomarkers, previously described, can be useful in monitoring the current state of the disease, the effectiveness of the treatment, and possibly predict the progression. However, currently the single ideal biomarker displaying high specificity and sensitivity for discriminating and monitoring this disease has not been determined. Thus, the combination of different biomarkers could be more advantageous than single biomarkers [93]. This would provide a more accurate panorama of the state of periodontal disease.

Classic methods for periodontitis diagnosis as the inspection and the palpation by the specialist can be relatively inaccurate. Additionally, the use of periodontal probes, and radiography could only provide information about previous periodontal damage rather than the current state [93]. Thus, biomarkers have been proposed as complementary methods to defeat the mentioned limitations monitoring the clinical response to an intervention and future risk [95].

Desirable's characteristics in test using biomarkers in periodontitis are easy to perform, rapid, and low cost, which could allow clinicians to perform early diagnosis and more effective personalized treatment.

Different factors are involved in the development of periodontitis, and a complex interaction between bacteria and immune system is observed. Additionally, periodontitis has been linked to at least 43 systemic diseases [96]. Thus, it is important to be careful when interpreting the results of biomarker tests because different factors could have a confounding impact on potential biomarkers [97]. Additionally, further large-scale studies are needed to prove specificity and sensitivity of the biomarkers analyzed in periodontitis and for utilization in routine clinical practice in the future.

5. Conclusions

Currently, a number of biomarkers have been sought for the detection of periodontal disease, but so far an ideal biomarker has not been found that helps early detection of the disease; perhaps the combination of several is the most appropriate.

The search for biomarkers continues, we suggest for further studies in search of new biomarkers, it should be consider having a larger sample size, a random source and keep a follow-up.

6. Future recommendations

Periodontal disease is already a very common problem in many countries; due to the above, the monitoring and reduction of the progress of periodontitis through surveillance and health promotion are part of the national health goal of countries like the United States [98].

Due to this, there has been an exhaustive search in recent years of biomarkers obtained from various sources, with saliva being the most used; however, we believe that new studies should include groups of patients with gingivitis on a daily basis, since this is considered an intermediate phase in which the patient can (if he/she carries out good dental hygiene and continues the treatment) stop the development of periodontitis [42], so that limit levels of these biomarkers may be detected.

In addition to this, numerous studies have shown so far that among the best options for biomarkers are proteins such as IL-1β, MMP-8, and ICTP.

From our point of view, we should also include and explore molecules such as miRNAs and other noncoding RNAs such as lncRNA and circRNA, in addition to the classical molecules that are already known to directly participate in the development of inflammatory pathology, since the study of these molecules could yield new perspectives on the development and progression of periodontal disease, which at some point may have important applications as biomarkers with leading activity in the development and manifestation of periodontitis.

Acknowledgements

We would like to appreciate the assistance of Ojeda Verdugo Einer Isaac, MD for providing technical editing and proofreading to improve the manuscript.

Conflict of interest

The authors declare no conflict of interest, financial, or otherwise.

Author details

Javier González-Ramírez[1,2*], Nicolás Serafín-Higuera[2,3],
Marina Concepción Silva Mancilla[3], Gustavo Martínez-Coronilla[4],
Jesús Famanía-Bustamante[3] and Ana Laura López López[1]

1 School of Nursing Campus Mexicali, Autonomous University of Baja California, Mexicali, Baja California, Mexico

2 Cell Biology Laboratory, Health Sciences Unit, Autonomous University of Baja California, Mexicali, Baja California, Mexico

3 School of Dentistry Campus Mexicali, Autonomous University of Baja California, Mexicali, Baja California, Mexico

4 Medical School Campus Mexicali, Autonomous University of Baja California, Mexicali, Baja California, Mexico

*Address all correspondence to: javier.gonzalez.ramirez@uabc.edu.mx

IntechOpen

References

[1] Trejo CSF, Cortés EM, Reyes LPF, Rodríguez JCM, Cisneros VO. Nivel de autocuidado y enfermedades bucales más frecuentes en pacientes de una clínica universitaria. Revista Iberoamericana de Ciencias de la Salud. 2017;**6**(12):1-18. DOI: 10.23913/rics.v6i12.52

[2] Yucel-Lindberg T, Båge T. Inflammatory mediators in the pathogenesis of periodontitis. Expert Reviews in Molecular Medicine. 2013;**15**:e7, 1-e7,22. DOI: 10.1017/erm.2013.8

[3] Camargo Ortega VR, Bravo López LD, Visoso Salgado A, Mejia Sanchez F, Castillo Cadena J. Polymorphisms in glutathione S-transferase M1, T1, and P1 in patients with chronic periodontitis: A pilot study. International Scholarly Research Notices. 2014;**2014**:1-6. DOI: 10.1155/2014/135368

[4] Hernández-Monjaraz B, Santiago-Osorio E, Monroy-García A, Ledesma-Martínez E, Mendoza-Núñez VM. Mesenchymal stem cells of dental origin for inducing tissue regeneration in periodontitis: A mini-review. International Journal of Molecular Sciences. 2018;**19**(4):944. DOI: 10.3390/ijms19040944

[5] Pihlstrom BL, Michalowicz BS, Johnson NW. Periodontal diseases. The Lancet. 2005;**366**(9499): 1809-1820. DOI: 10.1016/S0140-6736(05)67728-8

[6] Demmer RT, Behle JH, Wolf DL, Handfield M, Kebschull M, Celenti R, et al. Transcriptomes in healthy and diseased gingival tissues. Journal of Periodontology. 2008;**79**(11):2112-2124. DOI: 10.1902/jop.2008.080139

[7] Torres Courchoud I, Pérez Calvo JI. Biomarcadores y práctica clínica. Anales del Sistema Sanitario de Navarra. 2016;**39**(1):5-8. DOI: 10.4321/S1137-6627/2016000100001

[8] Arango VSS. Biomarcadores para la evaluación de riesgo en la salud humana. Revista Facultad Nacional de Salud Pública. 2012;**30**(1):75-82

[9] Lawrence T, Gilroy DW. Chronic inflammation: A failure of resolution? International Journal of Experimental Pathology. 2007;**88**(2):85-94. DOI: 10.1111/j.1365-2613.2006.00507.x

[10] Birkedal-Hansen H. Role of cytokines and inflammatory mediators in tissue destruction. Journal of Periodontal Research. 1993;**28**(7):500-510. DOI: 10.1111/j.1600-0765.1993.tb02113.x

[11] Jabłońska-Trypuć A, Matejczyk M, Rosochacki S. Matrix metalloproteinases (MMPs), the main extracellular matrix (ECM) enzymes in collagen degradation, as a target for anticancer drugs. Journal of Enzyme Inhibition and Medicinal Chemistry. 2016;**31**(suppl 1):177-183. DOI: 10.3109/14756366.2016.1161620

[12] Cekici A, Kantarci A, Hasturk H, Van Dyke TE. Inflammatory and immune pathways in the pathogenesis of periodontal disease. Periodontology 2000. 2014;**64**(1):57-80. DOI: 10.1111/prd.12002

[13] Aleo JJ, Padh H, Subramoniam A. Possible role of calcium in periodontal disease. Journal of Periodontology. 1984;**55**(11):642-647. DOI: 10.1902/jop.1984.55.11.642

[14] Wang CW, McCauley LK. Osteoporosis and periodontitis. Current Osteoporosis Reports. 2016;**14**(6):284-291. DOI: 10.1007/s11914-016-0330-3

[15] Prakash AR, Indupuru K, Sreenath G, Kanth MR, Reddy AVS, Indira Y. Salivary alkaline phosphatase levels speak about association of smoking, diabetes and potentially malignant diseases? Journal of Oral and Maxillofacial Pathology:

JOMFP. 2016;**20**(1):66-70. DOI:
10.4103/0973-029X.180934

[16] Dabra S, Singh P. Evaluating the levels
of salivary alkaline and acid phosphatase
activities as biochemical markers for
periodontal disease: A case series. Dental
Research Journal. 2012;**9**(1):41-45. DOI:
10.4103/1735-3327.92942

[17] Penido MGMG, Alon US. Phosphate
homeostasis and its role in bone
health. Pediatric Nephrology (Berlin,
Germany). 2012;**27**(11):2039-2048.
DOI: 10.1007/s00467-012-2175-z

[18] Foster BL, Tompkins KA, Rutherford
RB, Zhang H, Chu EY, Fong H, et al.
Phosphate: Known and potential roles
during development and regeneration of
teeth and supporting structures. Birth
Defects Research. Part C, Embryo Today:
Reviews. 2008;**84**(4):281-314. DOI:
10.1002/bdrc.20136

[19] Biosse Duplan M, Coyac BR, Bardet
C, Zadikian C, Rothenbuhler A,
Kamenicky P, et al. Phosphate and
vitamin D prevent periodontitis in
X-linked hypophosphatemia. Journal of
Dental Research. 2016;**96**(4):388-395.
DOI: 10.1177/0022034516677528

[20] Galgut PN. The relevance of pH
to gingivitis and periodontitis. Journal
of the International Academy of
Periodontology. 2001;**3**(3):61-67

[21] Saini R, Marawar PP, Shete S,
Saini S. Periodontitis, a true
infection. Journal of Global Infectious
Diseases. 2009;**1**(2):149-150. DOI:
10.4103/0974-777X.56251

[22] Wang Y, Andrukhov O, Rausch-Fan
X. Oxidative stress and antioxidant
system in periodontitis. Frontiers in
Physiology. 2017;**8**:910, 1-910,13. DOI:
10.3389/fphys.2017.00910

[23] Ray PD, Huang BW, Tsuji Y. Reactive
oxygen species (ROS) homeostasis and
redox regulation in cellular signaling.

Cellular Signalling. 2012;**24**(5):981-990.
DOI: 10.1016/j.cellsig.2012.01.008

[24] Valavanidis A, Vlachogianni T,
Fiotakis C. 8-Hydroxy-2'-deoxyguanosine
(8-OHdG): A critical biomarker of
oxidative stress and carcinogenesis.
Journal of Environmental Science and
Health, Part C. 2009;**27**(2):120-139. DOI:
10.1080/10590500902885684

[25] Hienz SA, Paliwal S, Ivanovski S.
Mechanisms of bone resorption in
periodontitis. Journal of Immunology
Research. 2015;**2015**:615486. DOI:
10.1155/2015/615486

[26] Koizumi M, Takahashi S, Ogata E. B
one metabolic markers in
bisphosphonate therapy for skeletal
metastases in patients with breast
cancer. Breast Cancer. 2003;**10**(1):21-27.
DOI: 10.1007/BF02967621

[27] Chen FC. Alternative RNA
structure-coupled gene regulations in
tumorigenesis. International Journal of
Molecular Sciences. 2014;**16**(1):452-475.
DOI: 10.3390/ijms16010452

[28] Cao J. The functional role of long noncoding RNAs and epigenetics. Biological
Procedures Online. 2014;**16**(1):1-11. DOI:
10.1186/1480-9222-16-11

[29] Irwandi RA, Vacharaksa A. The role
of microRNA in periodontal tissue: A
review of the literature. Archives of Oral
Biology. 2016;**72**:66-74. DOI: 10.1016/j.
archoralbio.2016.08.014

[30] Luan X, Zhou X, Naqvi A, Francis M,
Foyle D, Nares S, et al. MicroRNAs and
immunity in periodontal health and
disease. International Journal of Oral
Science. 2018;**10**(3):24-24. DOI: 10.1038/
s41368-018-0025-y

[31] Du Souich P, García AG, Vergés J,
Montell E. Immunomodulatory
and anti-inflammatory effects of
chondroitin sulphate. Journal of Cellular
and Molecular Medicine. 2009;

13(8A):1451-1463. DOI: 10.1111/j.1582-4934.2009.00826.x

[32] Egea J, García AG, Verges J, Montell E, López MG. Antioxidant, antiinflammatory and neuroprotective actions of chondroitin sulfate and proteoglycans. Osteoarthritis and Cartilage. 2010;**18**:S24-S27. DOI: 10.1016/j.joca.2010.01.016

[33] Chaturvedi P, Singh AP, Batra SK. Structure, evolution, and biology of the MUC4 mucin. FASEB Journal: Official Publication of the Federation of American Societies for Experimental Biology. 2008;**22**(4):966-981. DOI: 10.1096/fj.07-9673rev

[34] Mejías-Luque R, Lindén SK, Garrido M, Tye H, Najdovska M, Jenkins BJ, et al. Inflammation modulates the expression of the intestinal mucins MUC2 and MUC4 in gastric tumors. Oncogene. 2010;**29**(12):1753-1762. DOI: 10.1038/onc.2009.467

[35] Humphrey SP, Williamson RT. A review of saliva: Normal composition, flow, and function. Journal of Prosthetic Dentistry. 2001;**85**(2):162-169. DOI: 10.1067/mpr.2001.113778

[36] Kumar B, Kashyap N, Avinash A, Chevvuri R, Sagar MK, Shrikant K. The composition, function and role of saliva in maintaining oral health: A review. International Journal of Contemporary Dental and Medical Reviews. 2017; Article ID 011217: 1-6. DOI: 10.15713/ins.ijcdmr.121

[37] Al-Maskari AY, Al-Maskari MY, Al-Sudairy S. Oral manifestations and complications of diabetes mellitus: A review. Sultan Qaboos University Medical Journal. 2011;**11**(2):179-186

[38] Yoshizawa JM, Schafer CA, Schafer JJ, Farrell JJ, Paster BJ, Wong DTW. Salivary biomarkers: Toward

future clinical and diagnostic utilities. Clinical Microbiology Reviews. 2013;**26**(4):781-791. DOI: 10.1128/CMR.00021-13

[39] Malamud D. Saliva as a diagnostic fluid. Dental Clinics of North America. 2011;**55**(1):159-178. DOI: 10.1016/j.cden.2010.08.004

[40] Javaid MA, Ahmed AS, Durand R, Tran SD. Saliva as a diagnostic tool for oral and systemic diseases. Journal of Oral Biology and Craniofacial Research. 2016;**6**(1):66-75. DOI: 10.1016/j.jobcr.2015.08.006

[41] Gorrel C, Andersson S, Verhaert L. Periodontal disease. In: Gorrel C, Andersson S, Verhaert L, editors. Veterinary Dentistry for the General Practitioner. 2nd ed. W.B. Saunders; 2013. pp. 97-119

[42] Informed Health Online. Cologne, Germany: Institute for Quality and Efficiency in Health Care (IQWiG); 2006. Gingivitis and periodontitis: Overview. 2011 [Updated 2014 Jun 18]. Available from: https://www.ncbi.nlm.nih.gov/books/NBK279593/

[43] Ebersole JL, Nagarajan R, Akers D, Miller CS. Targeted salivary biomarkers for discrimination of periodontal health and disease(s). Frontiers in Cellular and Infection Microbiology. 2015;**5**:62-73. DOI: 10.3389/fcimb.2015.00062

[44] Ebersole JL, Schuster JL, Stevens J, Dawson 3rd D, Kryscio RJ, Lin Y, Thomas MV, Miller CS. Patterns of salivary analytes provide diagnostic capacity for distinguishing chronic adult periodontitis from health. Journal of Clinical Immunology, 2013;**33**(1):271-279. DOI: 10.1007/s10875-012-9771-3

[45] Liukkonen J, Gürsoy UK, Pussinen PJ, Suominen AL, Könönen E. Salivary concentrations of interleukin (IL)-1β, IL-17A, and IL-23 vary in relation

to periodontal status. Journal of Periodontology. 2016;**87**(12):1484-1491. DOI: 10.1902/jop.2016.160146

[46] Rathnayake N, Åkerman S, Klinge B, Lundegren N, Jansson H, Tryselius Y, et al. Salivary biomarkers of oral health—A cross-sectional study. Journal of Clinical Periodontology. 2013;**40**(2):140-147. DOI: 10.1111/jcpe.12038

[47] Sánchez GA, Miozza VA, Delgado A, Busch L. Salivary IL-1β and PGE2 as biomarkers of periodontal status, before and after periodontal treatment. Journal of Clinical Periodontology. 2013;**40**(12):1112-1117. DOI: 10.1111/jcpe.12164

[48] Yue Y, Liu Q, Xu C, Loo WTY, Wang M, Wen G, et al. Comparative evaluation of cytokines in gingival crevicular fluid and saliva of patients with aggressive periodontitis. The International Journal of Biological Markers. 2013;**28**(1):108-112. DOI: 10.5301/JBM.5000014

[49] Oh H, Hirano J, Takai H, Ogata Y. Effects of initial periodontal therapy on interleukin-1β level in gingival crevicular fluid and clinical periodontal parameters. Journal of Oral Science. 2015;**57**(2):67-71. DOI: 10.2334/josnusd.57.67

[50] Morelli T, Stella M, Barros SP, Marchesan JT, Moss KL, Kim SJ, et al. Salivary biomarkers in a biofilm overgrowth model. Journal of Periodontology. 2014;**85**(12):1770-1778. DOI: 10.1902/jop.2014.140180

[51] Azuma MM, Samuel RO, Gomes-Filho JE, Dezan-Junior E, Cintra LTA. The role of IL-6 on apical periodontitis: A systematic review. International Endodontic Journal. 2014;**47**(7):615-621. DOI: 10.1111/iej.12196

[52] Ebersole JL, Kirakodu S, Novak MJ, Stromberg AJ, Shen S, Orraca L,

et al. Cytokine gene expression profiles during initiation, progression and resolution of periodontitis. Journal of Clinical Periodontology. 2014;**41**(9): 853-861. DOI: 10.1111/jcpe.12286

[53] Scarel-Caminaga R, Trevilatto P, Souza A, B Brito R, Line SRP. Investigation of an IL-2 polymorphism in patients with different levels of chronic periodontitis. Journal of Clinical Periodontology. 2002;**29**(7):587-591. DOI: 10.1034/j.1600-051x.2002.290701.x

[54] Gupta M, Chaturvedi R, Jain A. Role of monocyte chemoattractant protein-1 (MCP-1) as an immune-diagnostic biomarker in the pathogenesis of chronic periodontal disease. Cytokine. 2013;**61**(3):892-897. DOI: 10.1016/j.cyto.2012.12.012

[55] Nisha KJ, Suresh A, Anilkumar A, Padmanabhan S. MIP-1α and MCP-1 as salivary biomarkers in periodontal disease. The Saudi Dental Journal. 2018;**30**(4):292-298. DOI: 10.1016/j.sdentj.2018.07.002

[56] Syndergaard B, Al-Sabbagh M, Kryscio RJ, Xi J, Ding X, Ebersole JL, et al. Salivary biomarkers associated with gingivitis and response to therapy. Journal of Periodontology. 2014;**85**(8):e295-e303. DOI: 10.1902/jop.2014.130696

[57] Eivazi M, Falahi N, Eivazi N, Eivazi MA, Raygani AV, Rezaei F. The effect of scaling and root planning on salivary TNF-α and IL-1α concentrations in patients with chronic periodontitis. The Open Dentistry Journal. 2017;**11**:573-580. DOI: 10.2174/1874210601711010573

[58] Ng PYB, Donley M, Hausmann E, Hutson AD, Rossomando EF, Scannapieco FA. Candidate salivary biomarkers associated with alveolar bone loss: Cross-sectional and in vitro studies. FEMS Immunology and Medical

Microbiology. 2007;**49**(2):252-260. DOI: 10.1111/j.1574-695X.2006.00187.x

[59] Franco C, Patricia H-R, Timo S, Claudia B, Marcela H. Matrix metalloproteinases as regulators of periodontal inflammation. International Journal of Molecular Sciences. 2017;**18**(2):440. DOI: 10.3390/ijms18020440

[60] Sapna G, Gokul S, Bagri-Manjrekar K. Matrix metalloproteinases and periodontal diseases. Oral Diseases. 2014;**20**(6):538-550. DOI: 10.1111/odi.12159

[61] Gursoy UK, Könönen E, Huumonen S, Tervahartiala T, Pussinen PJ, Suominen AL, et al. Salivary type I collagen degradation end-products and related matrix metalloproteinases in periodontitis. Journal of Clinical Periodontology. 2013;**40**(1):18-25. DOI: 10.1111/jcpe.12020

[62] Miricescu D, Totan A, Calenic B, Mocanu B, Didilescu A, Mohora M, et al. Salivary biomarkers: Relationship between oxidative stress and alveolar bone loss in chronic periodontitis. Acta Odontologica Scandinavica. 2014;**72**(1):42-47. DOI: 10.3109/00016357.2013.795659

[63] Borujeni S, Mayer M, Eickholz P. Activated matrix metalloproteinase-8 in saliva as diagnostic test for periodontal disease? A case-control study. Medical Micriobology and Immunology. 2015;**204**(6):665-672. DOI: 10.1007/s00430-015-0413-2

[64] Gupta N, Gupta ND, Gupta A, Khan S, Bansal N. Role of salivary matrix metalloproteinase-8 (MMP-8) in chronic periodontitis diagnosis. Frontiers of Medicine. 2015;**9**(1):72-76. DOI: 10.1007/s11684-014-0347-x

[65] Lira-Junior R, Öztürk VÖ, Emingil G, Bostanci N, Boström EA. Salivary and serum markers related to innate immunity in generalized aggressive periodontitis. Journal of Periodontology. 2017;**88**(12):1339-1347. DOI: 10.1902/jop.2017.170287

[66] Virtanen E, Yakob M, Tervahartiala T, Söder P-Ö, Andersson LC, Sorsa T, et al. Salivary MMP-13 gender differences in periodontitis: A cross-sectional study from Sweden. Clinical and Experimental Dental Research. 2017;**3**(5):165-170. DOI: 10.1002/cre2.76

[67] Mauramo M, Ramseier AM, Mauramo E, Buser A, Tervahartiala T, Sorsa T, et al. Associations of oral fluid MMP-8 with periodontitis in Swiss adult subjects. Oral Diseases. 2018;**24**(3):449-455. DOI: 10.1111/odi.12769

[68] Fiyaz M, Ramesh A, Ramalingam K, Thomas B, Shetty S, Prakash P. Association of salivary calcium, phosphate, pH and flow rate on oral health: A study on 90 subjects. Journal of Indian Society of Periodontology. 2013;**17**(4):454-460. DOI: 10.4103/0972-124X.118316

[69] Patel RM, Varma S, Suragimath G, Zope S. Estimation and comparison of salivary calcium, phosphorous, alkaline phosphatase and pH levels in periodontal health and disease: A cross-sectional biochemical study. Journal of Clinical and Diagnostic Research: JCDR. 2016;**10**(7):ZC58-ZC61. DOI: 10.7860/jcdr/2016/20973.8182

[70] Sevón L, Mäkelä M. A study of the possible correlation of high salivary calcium levels with periodontal and dental conditions in young adults. Archives of Oral Biology. 1990;**35**:S211-S212. DOI: 10.1016/0003-9969(90)90160-c

[71] Baliga S, Muglikar S, Kale R. Salivary pH: A diagnostic biomarker. Journal of Indian Society of Periodontology.

2013;**17**(4):461-465. DOI:
10.4103/0972-124X.118317

[72] Mishra D, Gopalakrishnan S,
Arun KV, Kumar TSS, Devanathan
S, Misra SR. Evaluation of salivary
levels of pyridinoline cross linked
carboxyterminal telopeptide of type
I collagen (ICTP) in periodontal
health and disease. Journal of
Clinical and Diagnostic Research.
2015;**9**(9):ZC50-ZC55. DOI: 10.7860/
jcdr/2015/12689.6498

[73] De Aguiar MCSM, Perinetti G,
Capelli J. The gingival crevicular
fluid as a source of biomarkers to
enhance efficiency of orthodontic
and functional treatment of
growing patients. BioMed Research
International. 2017;**2017**:1-7. DOI:
10.1155/2017/3257235

[74] Rahnama M, Czupkałło L, Kozicka-
Czupkałło M, Łobacz M. Gingival
crevicular fluid—Composition and
clinical importance in gingivitis and
periodontitis. Polish Journal of Public
Health. 2014;**124**(2):96-98. DOI:
10.2478/pjph-2014-0022

[75] Gupta G. Gingival crevicular
fluid as a periodontal diagnostic
indicator-I: Host derived enzymes and
tissue breakdown products. Journal of
Medicine and Life. 2012;**5**(4):390-397

[76] Becerik S, Öztürk VÖ, Atmaca
H, Atilla G, Emingil G. Gingival
crevicular fluid and plasma acute-
phase cytokine levels in different
periodontal diseases. Journal of
Periodontology. 2012;**83**(10):1304-
1313. DOI: 10.1902/jop.2012.110616

[77] Kinney JS, Morelli T, Oh M,
Braun TM, Ramseier CA, Sugai JV,
et al. Crevicular fluid biomarkers
and periodontal disease progression.
Journal of Clinical Periodontology.
2014;**41**(2):113-120. DOI: 10.1111/
jcpe.12194

[78] Branco-de-Almeida LS, Cruz-
Almeida Y, Gonzalez-Marrero Y,
Huang H, Aukhil I, Harrison P, et al.
Local and plasma biomarker profiles
in localized aggressive periodontitis.
JDR Clinical and Translational
Research. 2017;**2**(3):258-268. DOI:
10.1177/2380084417701898

[79] Lundmark A, Johannsen G,
Eriksson K, Kats A, Jansson L,
Tervahartiala T, et al. Mucin 4 and
matrix metalloproteinase 7 as novel
salivary biomarkers for periodontitis.
Journal of Clinical Periodontology.
2017;**44**(3):247-254. DOI: 10.1111/
jcpe.12670

[80] Khongkhunthian S, Kongtawelert
P, Ongchai S, Pothacharoen P, Sastraruji
T, Jotikasthira D, et al. Comparisons
between two biochemical markers
in evaluating periodontal disease
severity: A cross-sectional study. BMC
Oral Health. 2014;**14**(1):1-8. DOI:
10.1186/1472-6831-14-107

[81] Micó-Martínez P, García-Giménez
JL, Seco-Cervera M, López-Roldán A,
Almiñana-Pastor PJ, Alpiste-Illueca F, et al.
MiR-1226 detection in GCF as potential
biomarker of chronic periodontitis: A pilot
study. Medicina Oral, Patologia Oral y
Cirugia Bucal. 2018;**23**(3):e308-e314. DOI:
10.4317/medoral.22329

[82] Öngöz Dede F, Özden FO, Avcı
B. 8-Hydroxy-deoxyguanosine
levels in gingival crevicular fluid
and saliva in patients with chronic
periodontitis after initial periodontal
treatment. Journal of Periodontology.
2013;**84**(6):821-828. DOI: 10.1902/
jop.2012.120195

[83] Aruna G. Estimation of N-terminal
telopeptides of type I collagen in
periodontal health, disease and after
nonsurgical periodontal therapy
in gingival crevicular fluid: A
clinicobiochemical study. Indian Journal
of Dental Research. 2015;**26**(2):152-157.
DOI: 10.4103/0970-9290.159145

[84] Yu Z, Kastenmüller G, He Y, Belcredi P, Möller G, Prehn C, et al. Differences between human plasma and serum metabolite profiles. PLoS One. 2011;**6**(7):e21230. DOI: 10.1371/journal. pone.0021230

[85] Nile C, Apatzidou D, Raja Awang RA, P Riggio M, Kinane D, Lappin D. The effect of periodontal scaling and root polishing on serum IL-17E concentrations and the IL-17A:IL-17E ratio. 2016;**20**(9):2529-2537

[86] Boström EA, Kindstedt E, Sulniute R, Palmqvist P, Majster M, Holm CK, et al. Increased eotaxin and MCP-1 levels in serum from individuals with periodontitis and in human gingival fibroblasts exposed to pro-inflammatory cytokines. PLoS One. 2015;**10**(8):e0134608. DOI: 10.1371/journal.pone.0134608

[87] Sreeram M, Suryakar AN, Dani NH. Is non-surgical transpeptidase a biomarker for oxidative stress in periodontitis? Journal of Indian Society of Periodontology. 2015;**19**(2):150-154. DOI: 10.4103/0972-124X.149032

[88] Önder C, Kurgan Ş, Altıngöz SM, Bağış N, Uyanık M, Serdar MA, et al. Impact of non-surgical periodontal therapy on saliva and serum levels of markers of oxidative stress. Clinical Oral Investigations. 2017;**21**(6):1961-1969. DOI: 10.1007/s00784-016-1984-z

[89] Baltacıoğlu E, Yuva P, Aydın G, Alver A, Kahraman C, Karabulut E, et al. Lipid peroxidation levels and total oxidant/antioxidant status in serum and saliva from patients with chronic and aggressive periodontitis. Oxidative stress index: A new biomarker for periodontal disease? Journal of Periodontology. 2014;**85**(10):1432-1441. DOI: 10.1902/jop.2014.130654

[90] Nizam N, Meriç Gümüş P, Pitkänen J, Tervahartiala T, Sorsa T, Buduneli N. Serum and salivary matrix metalloproteinases, neutrophil elastase, myeloperoxidase in patients with chronic or aggressive periodontitis. Inflammation. 2014;**37**(5):1771-1778. DOI: 10.1007/s10753-014-9907-0

[91] Meschiari CA, Marcaccini AM, Santos Moura BC, Zuardi LR, Tanus-Santos JE, Gerlach RF. Salivary MMPs, TIMPs, and MPO levels in periodontal disease patients and controls. Clinica Chimica Acta. 2013;**421**:140-146. DOI: 10.1016/j.cca.2013.03.008

[92] Geyer PE, Holdt LM, Teupser D, Mann M. Revisiting biomarker discovery by plasma proteomics. Molecular Systems Biology. 2017;**13**(9):942-942. DOI: 10.15252/msb.20156297

[93] He W, You M, Wan W, Xu F, Li F, Li A. Point-of-care periodontitis testing: Biomarkers, current technologies, and perspectives. Trends in Biotechnology. 2018;**36**(11):1127-1144. DOI: 10.1016/j.tibtech.2018.05.013

[94] Gul SS, Douglas CWI, Griffiths GS, Rawlinson A. A pilot study of active enzyme levels in gingival crevicular fluid of patients with chronic periodontal disease. Journal of Clinical Periodontology. 2016;**43**(8):629-636. DOI: 10.1111/jcpe.12568

[95] Recker EN, Brogden KA, Avila-Ortiz G, Fischer CL, Pagan-Rivera K, Dawson DV, et al. Novel biomarkers of periodontitis and/or obesity in saliva—An exploratory analysis. Archives of Oral Biology. 2015;**60**(10):1503-1509. DOI: 10.1016/j.archoralbio.2015.07.006

[96] Slots J. Periodontitis: Facts, fallacies and the future. Periodontology 2000. 2017;**75**(1):7-23. DOI: 10.1111/prd.12221

[97] Lahdentausta L, Paju S, Mäntylä P, Buhlin K, Pietiäinen M, Tervahartiala

T, et al. Smoking confounds the
periodontal diagnostics using saliva
biomarkers. Journal of Periodontology.
2018; accepted/in press. DOI: 10.1002/
jper.18-0545

[98] Eke PI, Dye BA, Wei L, Slade GD,
Thornton-Evans GO, Borgnakke
WS, et al. Update on prevalence of
periodontitis in adults in the United
States: NHANES 2009 to 2012. Journal
of Periodontology. 2015;**86**(5):611-622

Chapter 3

Genetic Biomarkers in Periodontal Disease Diagnosis

Gurumoorthy Kaarthikeyan and Swarna Meenakshi

Abstract

Periodontitis is a chronic inflammatory disease with multifactorial etiology. The anaerobic bacteria have been implicated as the main etiological factor for periodontal destruction. Not all the individuals having the similar amount of plaque and calculus develop the periodontitis. Thus, the host susceptibility to periodontal pathogens plays a significant role in the etiopathogenesis of periodontitis. The genetic factor is the major determinant of the host susceptibility. There are contradictory results and varied results of the association of various genetic loci of different genes with periodontitis in different ethnic populations. This chapter will briefly discuss the various candidates' gene approach in understanding the etiopathogenesis of periodontitis. This chapter also throws some light on the relationship of the recent advances in genetic analysis like genome wide association studies, epigenetic regulation, and infectogenomics with periodontal destruction.

Keywords: gene polymorphisms, SNPs, periodontitis, genome wide association studies, infectogenomics, epigenetics

1. Introduction

The interplay among the immune system, microbiota, and lifestyle habits like smoking, alcoholism, stress, and diet that leads to constant changes in the host is regulated by genes. These genes encode immune receptors and various molecules involved in the signal transduction pathways that play an essential role in up regulation or down regulation of the immune response essentially the inflammatory reaction in response to a stimuli. Genetic research has focused on understanding how these responses work and also how these responses differ between different individuals. In addition to playing a role in health, the genetic factors also plays a major role in disease susceptibility. This review focuses on the genetic aspects of periodontal diseases wherein researchers are currently focusing on genetic evidences to explain the difference in susceptibility to periodontal disease in different individuals.

Although very prevalent, periodontal diseases are not evenly distributed across populations. Few people, who do not have much contributing local factors such as plaque and calculus, still develop severe destruction of bone whereas some do not develop severe forms of periodontal diseases in spite of having a very poor oral hygiene. This differential expression of periodontitis leads researchers to question if genetics and heritability played a major role. The first evidence that genetics played a role in periodontal diseases emerged in the 1990s. Schafer et al. postulated that a key determinant of whether individuals developed periodontitis or not was dependent on the way their bodies responded to the microbes [1]. Genetic factors and environmental factors determine the susceptibility to disease.

A biomarker is a substance that could indicate a biologic state and is an objective measure to evaluate the current and future disease activity. The National Institutes of Health Biomarkers Definitions Working Group in 1998 defined a biomarker as "a substance that is measured objectively and evaluated as an indicator of normal biologic processes, pathogenic processes, or pharmacologic responses to a therapeutic intervention." These biomarkers could be determined in various biological media like saliva, serum, and gingival crevicular fluid in health as well as disease. Generally, a combination of biomarkers is used in order to predict disease activity.

Genetic susceptibility to multifactorial diseases like periodontitis is usually due to several gene polymorphisms instead of a single, or few, gene mutations. Subtle variations in the genetic code may result in altered expression of the encoded proteins, thereby making individuals with genotypes more susceptible to a given disease.

The genetic link with the etiopathogenesis of periodontitis was started with the initial finding of association of composite genotype (Interleukin-1α and IL-1β) with chronic periodontitis in Caucasian population by Kornman et al. [2]. Following him, lot of studies conducted in different ethnic races linking the association of composite genotype with periodontitis. But the results were contradictory in nature. A variety of single nucleotide polymorphisms of various signaling factors, receptors, connective tissue components, enzymes involved in the host defense against the invading microbes have been reported by several researchers. Use of the genetic risk score could be useful in assessing the susceptibility to periodontitis. However, conflicting results have been reported because of the heterogeneticity of the studies. Different variations in frequency of some alleles in different populations have been observed.

2. Candidate gene approach

2.1 Interleukin-1

Interleukin-1 (IL-1) is a pro-inflammatory cytokine, which is encoded by IL-1 gene cluster at the chromosomal position 2q13–21. It is produced by inflammatory cells such as monocytes, macrophages, and dendritic cells, which play an important role in the regulation of immune and inflammatory responses to infections. It is composed of two molecules, IL-1α and IL-1β. The former regulates intracellular events while the latter acts as an extracellular protein. It plays a major role in the regulation of the inflammatory mechanisms. Studies by Lavu et al., Hao et al. have proposed that IL-1 cluster gene single nucleotide polymorphisms were associated with higher risk for periodontitis [3, 4]. Kornman et al. reported a relationship between IL-1α −889 and IL-1β +3954 and the severity of periodontal disease [2].

Kobayashi et al. demonstrated that Asians had a low carriage rate of IL-1α −889 R-allele compared to the other populations [5]. A meta-analysis by Mao et al., showed that IL-1β +3954 polymorphism increases the risk of periodontal disease [6]. Other authors like Amirisetty et al., Masamatti et al. suggested a strong association of IL-1β −511 and +3954 with chronic periodontitis in Indians [7, 8]. Whereas the study by Kaarthikeyan et al. did not find any significant association between interleukin-1β (+3954) polymorphism with chronic periodontitis in Indian population [9].

Karimbux et al. in their systematic review and meta-analysis studied 13 studies and found that IL-1α and IL-1β (IL-1α (−889) C > T, IL-1α (+4845) G > T, IL-1β

(+3954) C > T, could be a significant contribution to the risk of developing periodontitis [10]. Similarly, Yin et al. in their meta-analysis has found an association between IL-1α rs17561 and IL-1β rs 1143634 polymorphisms and periodontitis [11]. IL-1 gene cluster single nucleotide polymorphisms cannot be considered a significant risk factor for all populations. They seem to contribute to risk of periodontitis in Asian populations.

2.2 Interleukin-6

Interleukin-6 is produced during inflammation by T cells. It is encoded by the IL-6 gene localized on chromosome 7p21. Interleukin-6 is a potent bone resorbing cytokine. It activates and regulates the osteoclasts. Thus, this plays a major role in the susceptibility and progression of periodontal destruction. Zhang et al. found significant association between IL-6 −1363 G/T and IL-6R +48,892 A/C polymorphisms with periodontitis in Chinese population [12]. In a meta-analysis by Nikolopoulos et al. on cytokine gene polymorphisms such as IL-1α, IL-1β, IL-6, and TNF which included 53 studies, no significant association was detected between IL-6 and chronic periodontitis [13].

2.3 Interleukin-10

It is an anti-inflammatory cytokine expressed by T helper cells. It is encoded on gene at 1q31-q32. The major regions of interleukin-10 single nucleotide polymorphisms studied were −1082, −819, and −592. However, conflicting results have been obtained. Berglundh et al. found positive associations between IL-10 SNP and periodontitis in Swedish and Brazilian population [14]. Scarel-Caminaga et al. did not find any significant association in the Caucasian population [15].

2.4 TNF-α

It is a proinflammatory cytokine produced by macrophages. Gene localized at 6p21.3. A meta-analysis by Nikolopoulos et al., which based on 17 studies showed that there was no association of the TNF-α promoter −308G/A polymorphism with periodontitis while another meta-analysis by Song et al. which also included 17 studies found that TNF-α −308 A allele was associated with periodontitis in Brazilian, Asian, and Turkish populations [13]. Ding et al. in their meta-analysis based on 15 studies found an association between TNF-α SNP and periodontitis in Asian and Caucasian population [16]. Thus, the role of TNF-α SNP in the etiopathogenesis of periodontitis has to be explored with further studies.

2.5 TGF-β

It is a multifunctional cytokine that plays an important role in cellular differentiation, apoptosis and angiogenesis. It exists in three isoforms TGF-β1, β2, and β3. Cui et al. in their meta-analysis found significant association between TGF-β SNP and periodontitis in Asian population. However, few other studies by different authors did not show any association.

2.6 IFN-γ

Produced by natural killer cells. The gene is located on chromosome 12q24. Heidari et al. found an association between IFN-γ SNP in Iranian population, while Holla et al. did not find any significant association [17].

2.7 Vitamin D

Vitamin D and Vitamin D receptor are important mediators of bone metabolism. SNPs or dysfunction could lead to bone resorption. The gene encoding vitamin D is located on 12q12-q14.

Gross et al. in their study found that Fok1 polymorphism was associated with periodontitis. Brett et al. in their study found TaqI, BsmI, FokI and ApaI SNPs were associated with periodontitis [18]. Kaarthikeyan et al. did not find any significant association of VDR Taq1 polymorphism with periodontitis in south Indian population [19]. Mashhadiabbas et al. in their meta-analysis based on 38 studies found an association of vitamin D receptor BsmI, TaqI, FokI, and ApaI polymorphisms with periodontitis [20].

2.8 Matrix metalloproteinase and tissue inhibitor of matrix metalloproteinase

Matrix metalloproteinases (MMPs) are the key enzymes, which play a major role in the destruction of the collagenous and non-collagenous proteins of the connective tissue component. This is essential for maintaining the normal tissue homeostasis. To date, at least 26 members of MMPs have been identified. In periodontitis, this tissue homeostasis is altered with more destruction of connective tissue components and less inhibition by the TIMPs. Elevated levels of MMP-1, MMP-2, MMP-3, MMP-8, and MMP-9 have been detected in gingival crevicular fluid, peri-implant sulcular fluid, and gingival tissue of periodontitis patients. Thus, the genetic changes of the MMPs and TIMPs might play a role in the etiopathogenesis of periodontitis. According to Li et al., there was no significant association of MMP1, 8, 9, 12, 2, or 13 polymorphism with periodontitis. They did a meta-analysis of 17 studies [21]. Thus, the role of MMPs and TIMPs gene polymorphism with periodontitis has to be explored with further refined studies.

3. Genome wide association analysis

Rhodin et al. in their systematic analysis listed top genes NIN, ABHD12B, WHAMM, AP3B2, CPEB1, HGD, ZNF675, EMK1, TNFRSF10B, HTR4, WDR59, JDP2, OTOF, ANGEL2, etc. that showed evidence of association with severity of periodontitis and colonization of microorganisms [22]. GWAS is a recent development in the field of research. It highlights suggestive loci that could play an important role in periodontitis. However, the method is expensive and technique sensitive. Many GWAS in periodontitis has been carried out and has shown differential expression of varied genes [23–26].

4. Epigenetic modifications

Epigenetic modifications such as DNA methylation, histone modifications and RNA-associated silencing (micro RNA) play a role in susceptibility to disease. These modifications express or repress certain genes.

Loo et al. in their study showed that methylation of E-Cadherin and COX-2 was observed in periodontitis patients. Nahid et al. demonstrated the expression of miR-146a in infections caused by periodontopathic bacteria. Park et al. in their study observed that miRNA-132 played a major role in pathogenesis induced by P. Gingivalis. Several studies have reported the influence of various microRNAs especially miR-146a, let-7a, miR-196a, miR-499a, and miR-125a in susceptibility to chronic periodontitis [27–29]. Priyanka et al. in their study have found association of microRNA-125a and microRNA-499a polymorphisms with chronic periodontitis in south Indian population [30].

5. Infectogenomics

Infectogenomics refers to the association of the host genetic variants like single nucleotide polymorphisms with the composition of the microbial complexes in the host body. The recent meta-analysis by Nibali et al. has shown an association of 13 host genetic variants with the red/orange complex bacteria in periodontitis. The study by Divaris et al. has shown an association of two genetic loci (KCNK1 and DAB2IP) with high colonization of red complex bacteria. A more detailed knowledge of the human oral microbiome could provide more information on its association with host genetic variants [31, 32].

6. Conclusion

Although there are several studies that associate various candidate gene polymorphisms to periodontitis, till date there is not much clarity in the genetic susceptibility to the disease since there are a multitude of etiological factors and epigenetic factors that contribute to the susceptibility as well as severity of periodontal disease. Future research should focus on the multitude of genes, their multiple interactions and the epigenetic regulation during different stages of periodontal disease pathogenesis is required to fully understand the molecular mechanisms behind the etiopathogenesis of periodontitis.

Author details

Gurumoorthy Kaarthikeyan* and Swarna Meenakshi
Department of Periodontics, Saveetha Dental College and Hospitals, Saveetha Institute of Medical and Technical Sciences (SIMATS), Chennai, India

*Address all correspondence to: drkarthik79@yahoo.co.in

IntechOpen

References

[1] Shlafer S, Riep B, Griffen AL, Petrich A, Hubner J, Berning M, et al. Filifactor alocis—Involvement in periodontal biofilms. BMC Microbiology. 2010;**10**(66):1-13. DOI: 10.1186/1471-2180-10-66

[2] Kornman KS, Crane A, Wang HY, Giovlne FS, Newman MG, Pirk FW, et al. The interleukin-1 genotype as a severity factor in adult periodontal disease. Journal of Clinical Periodontology. 1997;**24**(1):72-77

[3] Lavu V, Venkatesan V, Venkata Kameswara Subrahmanya Lakkakula B, Venugopal P, Paul SF, Rao SR. Polymorphic regions in the interleukin-1 gene and susceptibility to chronic periodontitis: A genetic association study. Genetic Testing and Molecular Biomarkers. 2015;**19**(4):175-181

[4] Hao L, Li JL, Yue Y, Tian Y, Wang M, Loo WT, et al. Application of interleukin-1 genes and proteins to monitor the status of chronic periodontitis. The International Journal of Biological Markers. 2013;**28**(1):92-99. DOI: 10.5301/JBM.5000013

[5] Kobayashi T, Ito S, Kuroda T, Yamamoto K, et al. The interleukin-1 and Fcgamma receptor gene polymorphisms in Japanese patients with rheumatoid arthritis and periodontitis. Journal of Periodontology. 2007;**78**:2311-2318

[6] Mao M, Zeng XT, Ma T, He W, Zhang C, Zhou J. Interleukin-1α −899 (+4845) C→ T polymorphism increases the risk of chronic periodontitis: Evidence from a meta-analysis of 23 case–control studies. Gene. 2013;**532**(1):121-126

[7] Masamatti SS, Kumar A, Baron TK, Mehta DS, et al. Evaluation of interleukin-1B (+3954) gene polymorphism in patients with chronic and aggressive periodontitis: A genetic association study. Contemporary Clinical Dentistry. 2012;**3**:144-149

[8] Amirisetty R, Patel RP, Das S, Saraf J, Jyothy A, Munshi A. Interleukin 1ß (+3954, −511 and −31) polymorphism in chronic periodontitis patients from North India. 2015;**73**(5):343-347

[9] Karimbux NY, Jayakumar ND, Padmalatha O, Sheeja V, Sankari M, Anandan B. Analysis of the association between interleukin-1β (+3954) gene polymorphism and chronic periodontitis in a sample of the south Indian population. Indian Journal of Dental Research. 2009;**20**(1):37

[10] Kaarthikeyan G, Saraiya VM, Elangovan S, Allareddy V, Kinnunen T, Kornman KS, et al. Interleukin-1 gene polymorphisms and chronic periodontitis in adult whites: A systematic review and meta-analysis. Journal of Periodontology. 2012;**83**(11):1407-1419

[11] Yin WT, Pan YP, Lin L. Association between IL-1α rs17561 and IL-1β rs1143634 polymorphisms and periodontitis: A meta-analysis. Genetics and Molecular Research. 2016;**15**(1):1-8

[12] Zhang HY, Feng L, Wu H, Xie XD. The association of IL-6 and IL-6R gene polymorphisms with chronic periodontitis in a Chinese population. Oral Diseases. 2014;**20**(1):69-75

[13] Nikolopoulos GK, Dimou NL, Hamodrakas SJ, Bagos PG. Cytokine gene polymorphisms in periodontal disease: A meta-analysis of 53 studies including 4178 cases and 4590 controls. Journal of Clinical Periodontology. 2008;**35**(9):754-767

[14] Berglundh T, Donati M, Hahn-Zoric M, Hanson LÅ, Padyukov L. Association of the −1087 IL-10 gene polymorphism

with severe chronic periodontitis in Swedish Caucasians. Journal of Clinical Periodontology. 2003;**30**(3):249-254

[15] Scarel Caminaga RM, Trevilatto PC, Souza AP, Brito RB, Camargo LE, Line SR. Interleukin 10 gene promoter polymorphisms are associated with chronic periodontitis. Journal of Clinical Periodontology. 2004;**31**(6):443-448

[16] Ding C, Ji X, Chen X, Xu Y, Zhong L. TNF-α gene promoter polymorphisms contribute to periodontitis susceptibility: Evidence from 46 studies. Journal of Clinical Periodontology. 2014;**41**(8):748-759

[17] Holla LI, Hrdlickova B, Linhartova P, Fassmann A. Interferon-γ + 874A/T polymorphism in relation to generalized chronic periodontitis and the presence of periodontopathic bacteria. Archives of Oral Biology. 2011;**56**(2):153-158

[18] Gross C, Krishnan AV, Malloy PJ, Eccleshall TR, Zhao XY, Feldman D. The vitamin D receptor gene start codon polymorphism: A functional analysis of FokI variants. Journal of Bone and Mineral Research. 1998;**13**(11):1691-1699

[19] Kaarthikeyan G, Jayakumar ND, Padmalatha O, Varghese S, Anand B. Analysis of association of TaqI VDR gene polymorphism with the chronic periodontitis in Dravidian ethnicity. Indian Journal of Human Genetics. 2013;**19**(4):465

[20] Mashhadiabbas F, Neamatzadeh H, Nasiri R, Foroughi E, Farahnak S, Piroozmand P, et al. Association of vitamin D receptor BsmI, TaqI, FokI, and ApaI polymorphisms with susceptibility of chronic periodontitis: A systematic review and meta-analysis based on 38 case–control studies. Dental Research Journal. 2018;**15**(3):155

[21] Li W, Zhu Y, Singh P, Ajmera DH, Song J, Ji P. Association of common variants in MMPs with periodontitis risk. Disease Markers. 2016;**2016**:1-20

[22] Rhodin K, Divaris K, North KE, Barros SP, Moss K, Beck JD, et al. Chronic periodontitis genome-wide association studies: Gene-centric and gene set enrichment analyses. Journal of Dental Research. 2014;**93**(9):882-890

[23] Hong KW, Shin MS, Ahn YB, Lee HJ, Kim HD. Genomewide association study on chronic periodontitis in Korean population: Results from the Yangpyeong health cohort. Journal of Clinical Periodontology. 2015;**42**(8):703-710

[24] Divaris K, Monda KL, North KE, et al. Exploring the genetic basis of chronic periodontitis: A genome-wide association study. Human Molecular Genetics. 2013;**22**(11):2312-2324

[25] Sanders AE, Sofer T, Wong Q, Kerr KF, Agler C, Shaffer JR, et al. Chronic periodontitis genome-wide association study in the Hispanic community health study/study of Latinos. Journal of Dental Research. 2017;**96**(1):64-72

[26] Offenbacher S, Divaris K, Barros SP, Moss KL, Marchesan JT, Morelli T, et al. Genome-wide association study of biologically informed periodontal complex traits offers novel insights into the genetic basis of periodontal disease. Human Molecular Genetics. 2016;**25**(10):2113-2129

[27] Nahid MA, Rivera M, Lucas A, Chan EK, Kesavalu L. Polymicrobial infection with periodontal pathogens specifically enhances microRNA miR-146a in ApoE−/− mice during experimental periodontal disease. Infection and Immunity. 2011;**79**(4):1597-1605

[28] Perri R, Nares S, Zhang S, Barros SP, Offenbacher S. MicroRNA modulation in obesity and periodontitis. Journal of Dental Research. 2012;**91**(1):33-38

[29] Kebschull M, Papapanou PN. Mini but mighty: Micro RNA s in the pathobiology of periodontal disease. Periodontology 2000. 2015 Oct;**69**(1):201-220

[30] Venugopal P, Lavu V, Rao SR, Venkatesan V. Association of microRNA-125a and microRNA-499a polymorphisms in chronic periodontitis in a sample south Indian population: A hospital-based genetic association study. Gene. 2017;**631**:10-15

[31] Nibali L, Di Iorio A, Onabolu O, Lin GH. Periodontal infectogenomics: Systematic review of associations between host genetic variants and subgingival microbial detection. Journal of Clinical Periodontology. 2016;**43**(11):889-900

[32] Divaris K, Monda KL, North KE, Olshan AF, Lange EM, Moss K, et al. Genome-wide association study of periodontal pathogen colonization. Journal of Dental Research. 2012;**91**(7_suppl):S21-S28

Chapter 4

Role of Radiographic Evolution: An Aid to Diagnose Periodontal Disease

Krishna Kripal and Aiswarya Dileep

Abstract

In periodontics, the main purpose of radiography is to detect the level of the alveolar bone including the pattern and extent of loss of the bone. Measurements which are of linear from the cement-enamel junction to the crest of the alveolar bone and from the cement enamel junction to the bone defect base are commonly used to measure the bone height and bone defects. In radiographs, the periodontal ligament space, lamina dura and periapical region are seen and also helpful in identifying risk, such as calculus and dislodged restorations. Radiographs can provide information for proper diagnosis and treatment planning, which can provide information for the assessment of accurate treatment outcomes.

Keywords: computed tomography, cone beam computed tomography, tuned aperture computed tomography, magnetic resonance imaging, ultrasonography

1. Introduction

Ever since the discovery of X-rays by Wilhelm Conrad Roentgen in 1895, the diagnostic capabilities of medical and dental professions has been revolutionized and forever changed the practice of medicine and dentistry. Substantial advances in X-ray generator and X-ray detector technology have resulted in significant dose reductions and improved image quality. These advances in oral radiography have transformed into meaningful clinical applications improving the way we prevent, diagnose and treat periodontal disease [1–3].

In periodontics, the main purpose of radiography is to detect the level of the alveolar bone including the pattern and extent of bone loss. Measurements which are of linear from the cement enamel junction to the crest of alveolar bone and from the cement enamel junction to the osseous defect base are commonly used to measure crestal bone levels and osseous defects [4–7]. In radiographs, the periodontal ligament space, lamina dura and periapical region are evident and also useful in identifying risk factors, such as calculus and defective restorations [8].

Radiographs are valuable for diagnosis of periodontal disease, estimation of severity, determination of prognosis, and evaluation of treatment outcome. However, radiographs are an adjunct to the clinical examination, not a substitute for it. Radiographs demonstrate changes in calcified tissue; they do not reveal current cellular activity but rather reflect the effects of past cellular experience on the bone and roots.

Radiographs can provide critical information for diagnosis and treatment planning, which can also serve as baseline information for the assessment of treatment outcomes [9–11].

IntechOpen

Periodontist need to understand the strength and weakness of diagnostic imaging and way the cost and benefits of the test before prescribing it. Prescribing the appropriate type and the number of radiographs is critical for optimizing the impact of radiographs on treatment out comes.

The adaption of imaging which is digital as a modality of radiographic assessment of the feature, according to scientific evidence, has the potential to change the way to see the periodontal tissues. There is a little doubt that future periodontist will be using as advanced imaging modalities, either directly or indirectly [12].

2. Normal interdental bone

Evaluation of bone changes in periodontal disease is based mainly on the appearance of the interdental bone because the relatively dense root structure obscures the facial and lingual bony plates. The bone which is present interdentally normally is seen as a radiopaque line beside the periodontal ligament (PDL) and at the bone margin, called as the lamina dura. Because this thin line represents the cortical bone which lining the socket, and change in the angulation of the beam produce changes in its appearance [13, 14].

Crest of the interdental bone normally vary according to the convexity of the proximal tooth surfaces and the level of the cementoenamel junction (CEJ) of the approximating teeth. The faciolingual diameter of the bone is related to the width of the proximal root surface. The angulation of the crest of the interdental septum is generally parallel to a line between the CEJs of the approximating teeth. When there is a difference in the level of the CEJs, the crest of the interdental bone appears angulated rather than horizontal [15] (**Figure 1**).

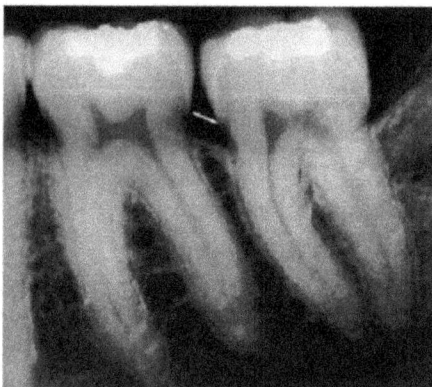

Figure 1.
Crest of interdental bone normally parallel to a line drawn between the cementoenamel junction of adjacent teeth (arrow). Note also the radiopaque lamina dura around the roots and interdental bone.

3. Radiographic techniques

In conventional radiographs, periapical and bite-wing projections offer the most diagnostic information and are most commonly used in the evaluation of periodontal disease. To properly and accurately depict periodontal bone status, proper techniques of exposure and processing are required. The bone level, pattern of bone destruction, PDL space width, as well as the radiodensity, trabecular pattern, and marginal contour of the interdental bone, vary by modifying exposure and development time, type of film, and X-ray angulation. Standardized, reproducible techniques are required to obtain reliable radiographs for pretreatment and posttreatment comparisons. Prichard put forward the following four criteria for the determination of adequate angulation of periapical radiographs [16–18]:

1. The periapical radiograph should have the ability to show the cusps of molars with occlusal surface.

2. Enamel and pulp chambers should be seen and distinct.

3. Open interproximal spaces.

4. Contacts between the adjacent teeth should not overlap unless teeth are out of line. For periapical radiographs, the long-cone paralleling technique most accurately projects the alveolar bone level.

The bisection-of-the-angle technique elongates the projected image, making the bone margin appear closer to the crown; the level of the facial bone is distorted more than that of the lingual. Inappropriate horizontal angulation results in tooth overlap, changes the shape of the interdental bone image, alters the radiographic width of the PDL space and the appearance of the lamina dura, and may distort the extent of furcation involvement [19].

Periapical radiographs frequently do not reveal the correct relationship between the alveolar bone and the CEJ. This is particularly true in cases in which a shallow palate or floor of the mouth does not allow ideal placement of the periapical film. Bite-wing projections offer an alternative that better images periodontal bone levels. For bite-wing radiographs, the film is placed behind the crowns of the upper and lower teeth parallel to the long axis of the teeth. The X-ray beam is directed

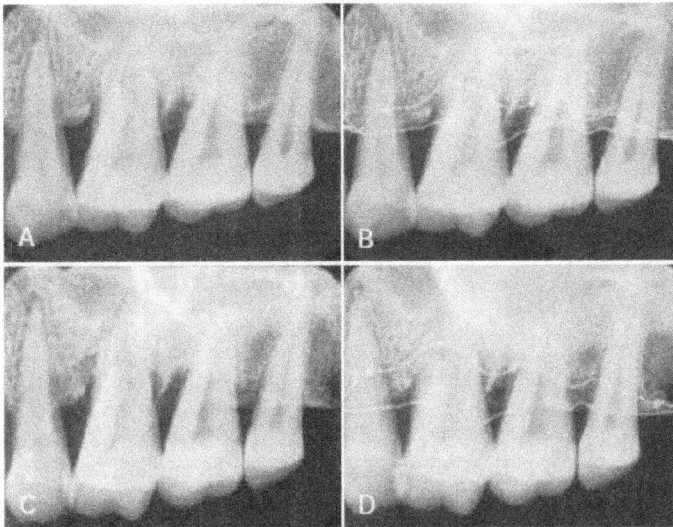

Figure 2.
Comparison of long-cone paralleling and bisection-of-the-angle techniques. (A) Long-cone paralleling technique, radiograph of dried specimen. (B) Long-cone paralleling technique, same specimen as A. Smooth wire is on margin of the facial plate and knotted wire is on the lingual plate to show their relative positions. (C) Bisection-of-the angle technique, same specimen as A and B. (D) Bisection of the-angle technique, same specimen. Both bone margins are shifted toward the crown, the facial margin (smooth wire) more than the lingual margin (knotted wire), creating the illusion that the lingual bone margin has shifted apically.

through the contact areas of the teeth and perpendicular to the film. Thus the projection geometry of the bite-wing films allows the evaluation of the relationship between the interproximal alveolar crest and the CEJ without distortion. If the periodontal bone loss is severe and the bone level cannot be visualized on regular bite-wing radiographs, films can be placed vertically to cover a larger area of the jaws. More than two vertical bite-wing films might be necessary to cover all the interproximal spaces of the area of interest [20] (**Figure 2**).

4. Bone destruction in periodontal disease

Early destructive changes of bone that do not remove sufficient mineralized tissue cannot be captured on radiographs. Therefore slight radiographic changes of the periodontal tissues suggest that the disease has progressed beyond its earliest stages. The earliest signs of periodontal disease must be detected clinically [16].

4.1 Bone loss

The radiographic image tends to underestimate the severity of bone loss. The difference between the alveolar crest height and the radiographic appearance ranges from 0 to 1.6 mm, mostly accounted for by X-ray angulation [21].

4.1.1 Amount

Radiographs are an indirect method for determining the amount of bone loss in periodontal disease; they image the amount of remaining bone rather than the amount lost. The amount of bone lost is estimated to be the difference between the physiologic bone level and the height of the remaining bone. The distance from the CEJ to the alveolar crest has been analyzed by several investigators. Most studies, conducted in adolescents, suggest a distance of 2 mm to reflect normal periodontium; this distance may be greater in older patients [22].

4.1.2 Distribution

The distribution of bone loss is an important diagnostic sign. It points to the location of destructive local factors in different areas of the mouth and in relation to different surfaces of the same tooth [23].

5. Pattern of bone destruction

In periodontal disease the interdental bone undergoes changes that affect the lamina dura, crestal radiodensity, size and shape of the medullary spaces, and height and contour of the bone. Height of interdental bone may be reduced, with the crest perpendicular to the long axis of the adjacent teeth horizontal bone loss; or angular or arcuate defects angular, or vertical, bone loss; could form [24–26].

Radiographs do not indicate the internal morphology or depth of craterlike defects. Also, radiographs do not reveal the extent of involvement on the facial and lingual surfaces. Bone destruction of facial and lingual surfaces is masked by the dense root structure, and bone destruction on the mesial and distal root surfaces may be partially hidden by superimposed anatomy, such as a dense mylohyoid ridge. In most cases, it can be assumed that bone losses seen interdentally continue in either the facial or the lingual aspect, creating a troughlike lesion [27].

Dense cortical facial and lingual plates of interdental bone obscure destruction of the intervening cancellous bone. Thus a deep craterlike defect between the facial and lingual plates might not be depicted on conventional radiographs. To record the destruction of the cancellous bone which is present interproximally and radiographically, the cortical bone must be involved. A decrease of only 0.5–1.0 mm in the thickness of the cortical plate is sufficient to permit radiographic visualization of the destruction of the inner cancellous trabeculae. Interdental bone loss may continue facially and/or lingually to form a troughlike defect that could be difficult to appreciate radiographically. These lesions may terminate on the radicular surface or may communicate with the adjacent interdental area to form one continuous lesion [28].

6. Radiographic appearance of periodontal disease

6.1 Periodontitis

Radiographic changes in periodontitis follow the pathophysiology of periodontal tissue destruction and include the following [29]:

1. Fuzziness and disruption of lamina dura crestal cortication continuity is the earliest radiographic change in periodontitis and results from bone resorption activated by extension of gingival inflammation into the periodontal bone. Depicting these early changes depends greatly on the radiographic technique, as well as on morphological changes. No correlation was found between

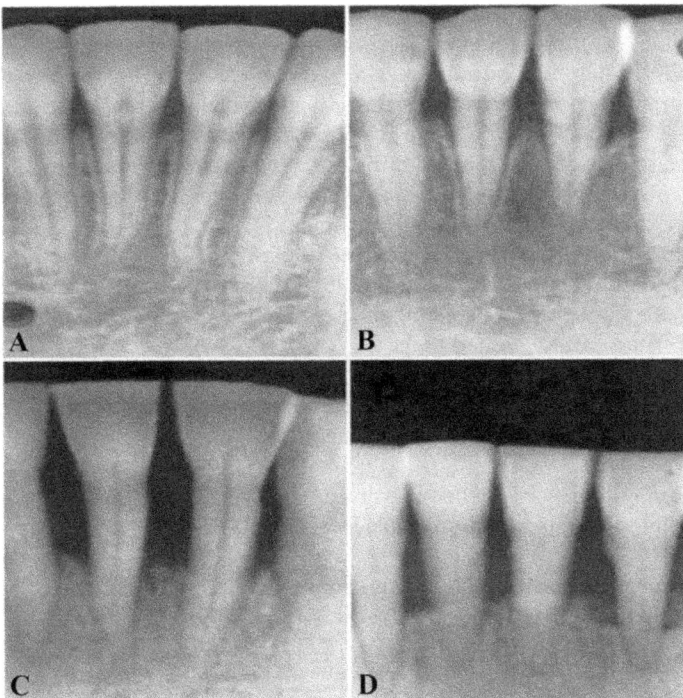

Figure 3.
Radiographic changes in periodontitis. (A) Normal appearance of interdental bone. (B) Fuzziness and a break in the continuity of the lamina dura at the crest of the bone distal to the central incisor (left). There are wedge-shaped radiolucent areas at the crest of the other interdental bone. (C) Radiolucent projections from the crest into the interdental bone indicate extension of destructive processes. (D) Severe bone loss.

lamina dura in radiographs and the presence or absence of clinical inflammation, bleeding on probing, periodontal pockets, or clinical attachment loss.
Therefore it can be concluded that the presence of an intact crestal lamina dura
may be an indicator of periodontal health (**Figure 3**).

2. Continued periodontal bone loss and widening of the periodontal space results
in a wedge-shaped radiolucency at the mesial or distal aspect of the crest. The
apex of the area is pointed in the direction of the root.

3. Subsequently, the destructive process extends across the alveolar crest, thus
reducing the height of the interdental bone. As increased osteoclastic activity
results in increased bone resorption along the endosteal margins of the medullary spaces, the remaining interdental bone can appear partially eroded.

4. The height of the interdental septum is progressively reduced by the extension
of inflammation and the resorption of bone.

5. Frequently a radiopaque horizontal line can be observed across the roots of a
tooth. This opaque line demarcates the portion of the root where the labial or
lingual bony plate has been partially or completely destroyed from the remaining bone-supported portion [30–32].

7. Furcation involvement

Definitive diagnosis of furcation involvement is made by clinical examination,
which includes careful probing with a specially designed probe (e.g., Nabers).
Radiographs are helpful, but root superimposition, caused by anatomic variations
and/or improper technique, can obscure radiographic representation of furcation
involvement. As a general rule, bone loss is greater than it appears in the radiograph. A tooth may present marked bifurcation involvement in one film but appear
to be uninvolved in another. Radiographs should be taken at different angles to
reduce the risk of missing furcation involvement [31].

The recognition of a large, clearly defined radiolucency in the furcation area is
easy to identify but less clearly defined radiographic changes are often overlooked.
To assist in the radiographic detection of furcation involvement, the following
diagnostic criteria are suggested [32]:

1. The radiographic change in the furcation area can be determined clinically,
especially if there is bone loss on adjacent roots.

2. Reduced radiodensity in the furcation area in which bony trabeculae outlines
are visible suggests furcation involvement of the teeth.

3. Whenever there is marked bone resorption in relation to a single molar root, it
can be assumed that the furcation of it is also involved (**Figure 4**).

8. Trauma from occlusion

Trauma from occlusion can produce visible changes radiographically in the
thickness of the lamina dura, morphology of the alveolar bone crest, width of the
PDL space, and density of the surrounding cancellous bone [31].

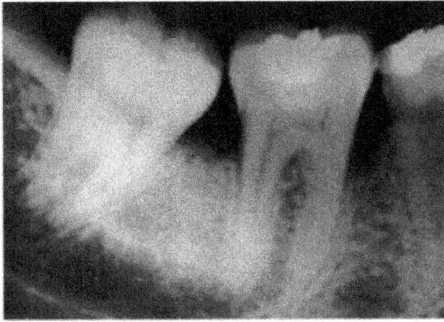

Figure 4.
Early furcation involvement suggested by fuzziness in the bifurcation of the mandibular first molar,
particularly when associated with bone loss on the roots.

Traumatic lesions manifest more clearly in faciolingual aspects because mesio-distally, the tooth has the added stability provided by the contact areas with adjacent teeth. Therefore slight variations in the proximal surfaces may indicate greater changes in the facial and lingual aspects. The radiographic changes listed next are not pathognomonic of trauma from occlusion and must be interpreted in combination with clinical findings, particularly tooth mobility, presence of wear facets, pocket depth, and analysis of occlusal contacts and habits [32].

The injury phase of trauma from occlusion produces a loss of the lamina dura that may be noted in apices, furcations, and marginal areas. This loss of lamina dura results in widening of the PDL space. The repair phase of trauma from occlusion results in an attempt to strengthen the periodontal structures to better support the increased loads. Radiographically, this is manifested by a widening of the PDL space, which may be generalized or localized [33].

9. Advanced procedures

9.1 Tomography

Tomography is a generic term formed by the Greek words "Tomo" (slice) and "Graph" (picture). So tomography refers to imaging by sections or sectioning, through the use of any kind of penetrating wave. A device used in tomography is called a tomography, while the image produced is a tomogram. Conventional film-based tomography, also called body section radiography is, a radiographic technique designed to image more clearly objects lying within a plane of interest. This is accomplished by blurring the images of structures lying outside the plane of interest through the process of motion "unsharpness."

In conventional medical X-ray tomography, sectional image is taken through a body by moving an X-ray source and the film in opposite directions during the exposure.

9.1.1 Main indications

The main clinical indicated to examine various facial structures:

- When a pathology is strongly suspected clinically, but plain films are negative.

- Preoperative assessment of jaw height, thickness and texture before inserting implants.

- Postoperative evaluation of implants.

- Tomography of sinuses.

- Tomography of facial bones, to study facial fractures.

- Evaluation of grossly comminuted facial fractures to determine all the fracture sites.

- Assessment of the extent of orbital blow-out fractures.

- The most commonly used radiographic modality for demonstrating maxillo-facial.

- Fractures are conventional radiography and it is still believed to be the most reliable.

- Diagnostic tool.

- As an additional investigation of the TMJ and condylar head particularly useful if.

- Patients are unable to open their mouths.

9.1.2 Advantages

- It gives a more precise evaluation of sinus pathologies, which are poorly visualized on.

- Routine radiography.

- Assessment of the size, position and extent of antral tumors.

- Sphenoid and ethmoidal sinuses are more clearly visualized.

- Similar optimum definition is obtainable on each slice.

9.1.3 Disadvantages

- The radiation dose to the patient may be high.

- The technique is time-consuming.

- A high level of cooperation is required as the patient has to remain in the same position throughout the investigation.

- Images appeared to be blurred.

10. Computed tomography (CT)

10.1 Introduction

In April of 1972 Godfrey Hounsfield a senior research scientist at EMI limited in Middlesex, England announced the invention of a revolutionary imaging technique.

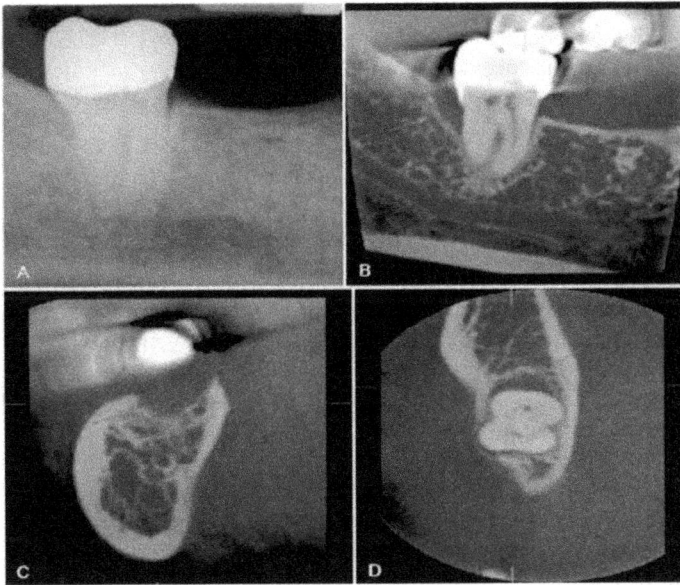

Figure 5.
Periapical radiograph (A) and sagittal (B), cross-sectional (C), and axial (D) cone-beam computed tomography (CBCT) sections of the mandibular right second molar. No pathology is detected on the periapical radiograph. However, CBCT images clearly illustrate a deep, vertical, three-wall defect on the distal surface of the mandibular right second molar (red arrow).

He referred this technique as computerized axial transverse scanning for which he received a Nobel prize in 1979. With this technique he was able to produce an axial cross sectional image of the head using a narrowly collimated, moving beam of X-rays [33, 34].

10.2 Cone beam computed tomography

In the last decade, cone-beam computed tomography (CBCT) has revolution-ized the field of oral and maxillofacial imaging. However, CBCT finds application in almost every diagnostic task of clinical dentistry, including evaluation of periodontal and periapical structures. CBCT offers many advantages over conventional radiography, including the accurate three-dimensional imaging of teeth and supporting structures. Although not recommended for every dental patient, CBCT avoids the problems of geometric superimposition and unpredictable magnification and can provide valuable diagnostic information in periodontal evaluation [35].

Periapical and bite-wing radiographs provide information mostly for the interdental bone. However, a three-wall defect that preserves the buccal and/or lingual cortices can be difficult to diagnose, and the buccal, lingual, and furcational periodontal bone levels are hard to evaluate in conventional radiographs. When clinical examination raises concerns for such areas, CBCT imaging can add diagnostic value [36–39] (**Figure 5**).

11. Advantages of CBCT in dentistry

Being considerably smaller, CBCT equipment has a greatly reduced physical footprint and is ~20–25% of the cost of conventional CT. CBCT provides images of high contrasting structures and is therefore particularly well-suited towards the imaging of osseous structures of the craniofacial area. The use of CBCT technology in clinical dental practice provides a number of advantages for maxillofacial imaging [40]. These include:

11.1 Rapid scan time

Because CBCT acquires all projection images in a single rotation, scan time is comparable to panoramic radiography. This is desirable because artifact due to subject movement is reduced. Computer time for dataset reconstruction however is substantially longer and varies depending on FOV, the number of basis images acquired, resolution and reconstruction algorithm and may range from ~1 to 20 minutes [41, 43].

11.2 Beam limitation

Collimation of the CBCT primary X-ray beam enables limitation of the X-radiation to the area of interest. Therefore an optimum FOV can be selected for each patient based on suspected disease presentation and region of interest. While not available on all CBCT systems, this functionality is highly desirable as it provides dose savings by limiting the irradiated field to fit the FOV.

11.3 Image accuracy

CBCT imaging produces images with sub-millimeter isotropic voxel resolution ranging from 0.4 mm to as low as 0.09 mm. Because of this characteristic, subsequent secondary (axial, coronal and sagittal) and MPR images achieve a level of spatial resolution that is accurate enough for measurement in maxillofacial applications where precision in all dimensions is important such as implant site assessment and orthodontic analysis [42].

11.4 Reduced patient radiation dose compared to conventional CT

Published reports indicate that the effective dose (E) varies for various full field of view CBCT devices from 29 to 477 µSv depending on the type and model of CBCT equipment and FOV selected patient positioning modifications (tilting the chin) and use of additional personal protection (thyroid collar) can substantially reduce dose by up to 40%. These doses can be compared more meaningfully to dose from a single digital panoramic exposure, equivalent CT dose, or the average natural background radiation exposure for Australia (1500 µSv) in terms of background equivalent radiation time (BERT). CBCT provides an equivalent patient radiation dose of 5–80 times that of a single film-based panoramic radiograph, 1.3–22.7% of a comparable conventional CT exposure or 7–116 days of background radiation.

11.5 Limitations of CBCT imaging

While there has been enormous interest, current CBCT technology has some limitations related to the "cone beam" projection geometry, detector sensitivity and resolution which is contrast. These parameters create an inherent image "noise" that reduces image clarity such that current systems are unable to record soft tissue contrast at the relatively low dosages applied for maxillofacial imaging.

Another factor that impairs CBCT image quality is image artifact three types of cone-beam-related artifacts:

Partial volume averaging: it occurs when the selected voxel resolution of the scan is greater than the spatial or contrast resolution of the object to be imaged.

Under sampling: under sampling can occur when too few basis projections are provided for the reconstruction. A reduced data sample leads to misregistration and sharp edges and noisier images because of aliasing, where fine striations appear in the image.

Cone-beam effect: the cone-beam effect is the major source of error, especially in the parts which are outside of the scan volume. Because of the divergence of as it rotates around the patient in a horizontal plane. The amount of data corresponds to the total amount of attenuation along a specific beam projection angle as the scanner completes an arc. Because the outer row pixels record less attenuation, whereas more information is recorded for objects projected onto the more central detector pixels, which results in image distortion, streaking artifacts.

11.6 Advantages of CBCT

1. CBCT has a scanning time which rapid as in comparison with panoramic radiography.

2. It allows reconstruction with proper three dimensional and display from an angle.

3. Its beam collimation makes limitation of X radiation to the area of interest.

4. Images clarity produces images ranging from 0.4 mm to as low as 0.076 mm.

5. Radiation dosage of patient is reduced (29–477 µSv) in comparison with conventional CT (~2000 µSv). Patient radiation dose is six times lesser than normal CT, as the exposure time is ~18 seconds.

6. The units of CBCT reconstruct the projection data to provide inter relational images in three orthogonal planes (axial, sagittal, and coronal).

7. Reformation which is multiplanar is possible by sectioning volumetric datasets nonorthogonally.

8. Multiplanar image can be "thickened" by increasing the number of voxels.

9. Volume rendering which is 3D is processed by direct or indirect technique.

10. The three positioning beams make patient positioning easy.

11. Reduced image artifacts: CBCT projection geometry, together with fast acquisition time, results in a low level of metal artifact in primary and secondary reconstructions.

11.7 Disadvantages

The only disadvantage is its cost. But considering the enormous benefits, this cost effect can be overlooked.

Indications of cone-beam computed tomography:

1. Assessment of the jaw which includes:

   • Pathological lesions which are bone and soft tissue;

- Periodontal assessment;

- Endodontic assessment;

- Alveolar ridge loss;

- Recognition of fractures and structural maxillofacial deformities;

- Assessment of the inferior alveolar nerve before extraction of mandibular third molar impactions.

12. Ultrasonography

Ultrasound imaging is easy to use for the detection of noninvasive and soft tissue related diseases. Ultrasonography utilizes sound waves for image production. The first major attempt at a practical application was made in search for the sunken Titanic in the North Atlantic in 1912. A few early attempts at applying US in medical diagnosis. Successful medical application began shortly after the war in the late 1940s and early 1950s. The vital ingredients are transducer, ultrasonic beam, a cathode ray tube or television monitor. The evolution of sonic imaging began slowly from a static one dimensional base (A-mode or amplitude mode), improved somewhat when a component of motion was added (TM-mode), made a giant leap forward with two dimensional imaging (B mode or brightness mode) and reached its current zenith with gray scale imaging. The phenomenon sound which are perceived is the result of changes which are periodic in the pressure of air against the eardrum. The periodicity of these changes ranging from 1500 to 20,000 cycles per second (hertz [Hz]). By definition, ultrasound has a periodicity >20 kHz. Thus it is distinguished from other waveforms which are mechanical simply by having a vibratory frequency more than the human audible range. Diagnostic ultrasonography (sonography), uses vibratory frequencies in the range of 1–20 MHz. Scanners which are used for sonography generate impulses which is electrical that are converted into sound waves which is of high frequency help of a transducer.

Transducer is a device that transform one form of energy into another-in this case, electrical energy can be converted into sonic energy. The most important part of the transducer is a thin piezoelectric crystal or material which is made up of a great number of dipoles arranged in a pattern of geometric. A dipole may be thought of as a distorted molecule which has two ends that appears to have a positive charge on one end and a negative charge on the other.

Applications of ultrasound in periodontics:

1. As diagnostic aid: ultrasonography probe gives a system of mapping for noninvasive procedure and calculate as well as record various measurements of subject's periodontal ligaments relative to a fixed point such as cementoenamel junction. This probe uses ultrasound to detect periodontal ligament and cement-enamel junction. This ultrasound probe records a series of measurements which is painless.

2. Assessment of periodontium: an ultrasonic scanner that functions at a frequency of 29 MHz has been used to detect the dimensional relationship between hard and soft structures of periodontium. This device also used to assess the gingival thickness before and after mucogingival surgery for gingival recession and to calculate the thickness of masticatory mucosa.

3. Detection of subgingival calculus: there are large number of subgingival calculus detection systems available found that dental surfaces may be determined separately by the tip oscillations analysis of an ultrasonic instrument, which has features of subgingival calculus detection.

4. Complete removal of dental plaque or the biofilm: removal of the bacterial plaque by means of the acoustic micro-streaming and cavitation effects of ultrasound. Many studies have shown that there is no statistically significant difference in the effectiveness of plaque removal using hand or motor driven instruments. It can also used for scaling in cases of necrotizing ulcerative lesions as this possess an action of lavage.

5. Removal of supra and subgingival calculus: cavitation effect liberates energy that can be able to remove the deposits. It is effective on the both supra and subgingival calculus, a direct contact between the vibrating tip and the calculus is needed.

6. Clearance of endotoxin and detoxification: the endotoxins are known to be fragments of bacterial cells and toxic products of bacteria and can be found in the root cementum or dentine, saliva and gingival crevicular fluid. Endotoxins are cytotoxic substances and can affect the immune system of the host. It is suggested that, for the successful treatment outcome, the infected dentine and altered cementum have to be removed. Recent studies have shown that endotoxin is superficially associated with the cementum and calculus. They can be easily removed by rinsing, brushing, lightly scaling, or polishing the root surface. Heat generated from magnetostrictive units may helpful in endotoxin removal or detoxification.

7. Curettage: ultrasound is effective for the debridement of the epithelial lining of periodontal pockets. A Morse scaler-shaped or rod-shaped ultrasonic instrument can be used. Ultrasonic instruments are found to be as effective as curettage done by hand instruments.

8. Osseous surgery: ultrasonic bone cutting surgery has been recently introduced as an alternative to the conventional techniques. Piezosurgery® is a new and innovative method that uses piezoelectric ultrasonic vibrations to do precise and safe osteotomies. Piezoelectric surgery uses a specifically engineered surgical instrument characterized by a surgical power that is three-times higher than normal ultrasonic instruments. The unique feature of this technique is that the cutting action occurs when tool is employed on the mineralized tissue, but stops when soft tissue is encountered. This technique can be used for preprosthetic surgery, sinus elevation procedure, implant placement as well as alveolar crest expansion.

13. Conclusions

Periapical radiographic examination should be part of each patient's periodontal evaluation and should be coupled with a detailed recording of pocket depths, gingival margin location, and bleeding on probing. Radiographic evaluation should be updated every 2 years. Periapical radiographs often underestimate the amount of periodontal bone loss, and early changes are usually not detected. Significant interdental bone loss can occur and may not be detectable on periapical radiographs because the density of the intact buccal and lingual or palatal bone plates obscure changes that occur as the result of periodontitis. Comparison of periapical radiographs of the same area taken at different times will only be reliable in documenting dramatic changes in bone levels since variations in angulation of the beam, placement of the film, and development of the image make accurate measurements taken over time very difficult and unreliable.

Recent use of three-dimensional radiographic techniques with CBCT gives a much more accurate picture of periodontal bone loss than do two-dimensional radiographs and will be more widely used as this technology becomes available in more clinics.

Conflict of interest

None.

Appendices and nomenclature

CEJ	cemento- enamel junction
PDL	periodontal ligament
TMJ	temperomandibular joint
CT	computed tomography
CBCT	cone beam computed tomography
FOV	field of view
MPR	multiplanar reformation
ARPANSA	australian radiation protection and nuclear safety agency
BERT	background equivalent radiation time
A MODE	amplitude mode
B MODE	brightness mode

Author details

Krishna Kripal* and Aiswarya Dileep
RajaRajeswari Dental College and Hospital, Bangalore, India

*Address all correspondence to: kripalkrishna@yahoo.com

IntechOpen

References

[1] Tomography at the US national library of medicine medical subject headings (MeSH) white and pharoh. p. 247

[2] Fuji N, Yamashiro M. Computed tomography for the diagnosis of facial fractures. Journal of Oral Surgery. 1981;**39**:735

[3] Kassel EE, Noyek AM, Cooper PW. CT in facial trauma. The Journal of Otolaryngology. 1983;**12**:2-5

[4] Abrahams JJ, Caceres C. Mandibular erosion from silastic implants: Evaluation with a dental CT software program. AJNR. American Journal of Neuroradiology. 1998;**19**:519-522

[5] Roithmann R, Kassell EE, Kirsch JC, Wortzman G, Abrahams JJ, Noyek AM. New radiographic techniques for detection of mandibular invasion by cancer. Operative Techniques in Otolaryngology-Head and Neck Surgery. 1993;**2**:149-154

[6] Yanagisawa K, Friedman C, Abrahams JJ. DentaScan imaging of the mandible and maxilla. Head & Neck. 1993;**14**:979-990

[7] Abrahams JJ, Olivario P. Odonotogenic cysts: Improved imaging with a dental CT software program. AJNR. American Journal of Neuroradiology. 1993;**14**:367-374

[8] Abrahams JJ, Berger S. Inflammatory disease of the jaw: Appearance on reformatted CT images. AJR. American Journal of Roentgenology. 1998;**170**:1085-1091

[9] Abrahams JJ, Glassberg RM. Dental disease: A frequently unrecognized cause of maxillary sinus abnormalities? AJR. American Journal of Roentgenology. 1995;**166**:1219-1223

[10] Abrahams JJ, Berger SB. Oral-maxillary sinus fistula oroantral fistula: Clinical presentation and evaluation with multiplanar CT. AJR. American Journal of Roentgenology. 1995;**165**:1273-1276

[11] Abrahams JJ, Levine B. Expanded applications of DentaScan: Multiplanar CT of the mandible and maxilla. The International Journal of Periodontics & Restorative Dentistry. 1990;**10**:464-467

[12] Abrahams JJ. Anatomy of the jaw revisited with a dental CT software program: Pictorial essay. AJNR. American Journal of Neuroradiology. 1993;**14**:979-990

[13] Lain S, Osaka F, Asanami S, Tomita O. Adenocytic carcinoma in computed tomography. Oral Surgery. 1980;**49**:552-555

[14] Ames JR, Johnson RP, Stevens EA. Computerized tomography in oral and maxillofacial surgery. Journal of Oral Surgery. 1980;**38**:145-149

[15] Cho PS, Johnson RH, Griffin TW. Cone-beam CT for radiotherapy applications. Physics in Medicine & Biology. 1995;**40**:1863-1883

[16] Spector L. Computer-aided dental implant planning. Dental Clinics of North America. 2008;**52**:761-775

[17] Razavi T, Palmer RM, Davies J. Accuracy of measuring the cortical bone thickness adjacent to dental implants using cone beam computed tomography. Clinical Oral Implants Research. 2010;**21**:718-725

[18] Lewis EL, Dolwick MF, Abramowicz S, Reeder SL. Contemporary imaging of the temporomandibular joint. Dental Clinics of North America. 2008;**52**:875-890

[19] Farman AG, Scarfe WC. The basics of maxillofacial cone beam computed

tomography. Seminars in Orthodontics. 2009;**15**:2-13

[20] Patel S, Dawood A, Ford TP, Whaites E. The potential applications of cone beam computed tomography in the management of endodontic problems. International Endodontic Journal. 2007;**40**:818-830

[21] Thomas SL. Application of cone-beam CT in the office setting. Dental Clinics of North America. 2008;**52**:753-759

[22] Jiomr. 22 (1): 2010. pp. 34-38

[23] Grant DG. Tomosynthesis: A three-dimensional radiographic imaging technique. IEEE Transactions on Biomedical Engineering. 1972;**19**:20-28

[24] Groenhius RA, Webber RL, Ruttimann UE. Computerized tomosynthesis of dental tissues. Oral Surgery, Oral Medicine, and Oral Pathology. 1983;**56**:206-214

[25] Webber RL, Horton RA, Tyndall DA, Ludlow JB. Tuned-aperture computed tomography (TACT1). Theory and application for three-dimensional dento-alveolar imaging. Dento Maxillo Facial Radiology. 1997;**26**:53-62

[26] Nair MK, Nair UP. Digital and advanced imaging in endodontics: A review. Journal of Endodontics. 2007;**33**:1-6

[27] Webber RL, Messura JK. An in vivo comparison of digital information obtained from tuned aperture computed tomography and conventional dental radiographic imaging modalities. Oral Surgery, Oral Medicine, Oral Pathology, Oral Radiology and Endodontology. 1999;**88**:239-247

[28] De Coene B, Hajnal JV, Gatehouse P, Longmore DB, White SJ, Oatridge A, et al. MR of the brain using fluid-attenuated inversion recovery (FLAIR) pulse sequences. American Journal of Neuroradiology. 1992;**13**(6):1555-1564

[29] Moseley ME, Cohen Y, Mintorovitch J, Chileuitt L, Shimizu H, Kucharczyk J, et al. Early detection of regional cerebral ischemia in cats: Comparison of diffusionand T2-weighted MRI and spectroscopy. Magnetic Resonance in Medicine. 1990;**14**(2):330-346

[30] Ridgway JP, Smith MA. A technique for velocity imaging using magnetic resonance imaging. The British Journal of Radiology. 1986;**59**(702):603-607

[31] Takashima S, Noguchi Y, Okumura T, Aruga H, Kobayashi T. Dynamic MR imaging in the head and neck. Radiology. 1993;**189**:813-821

[32] Asaumi J, Shigehara H, Konouchi H, et al. Assessment of carcinoma in the sublingual region based on magnetic resonance imaging. Oncology Reports. 2002;**9**:1283-1287

[33] Fischbein NJ, Noworolski SM, Henry RG, Kaplan MJ, Dillon WP, Nelson SJ. Assessment of metastatic cervical adenopathy using dynamic contrast-enhanced MR imaging. American Journal of Neuroradiology. 2003;**24**:301-311

[34] Noworolski SM, Fischbein NJ, Kaplan MJ, et al. Challenges in dynamic contrast-enhanced MRI imaging of cervical lymph nodes to detect metastatic disease. Journal of Magnetic Resonance Imaging. 2003;**17**:455-462

[35] Asaumi J, Yanagi Y, Hisatomi M, Matsuzaki H, Konouchi H, Kishi K. The value of dynamic contrast enhanced MRI in diagnosis of malignant lymphoma of the head and neck. European Journal of Radiology. 2003;**48**:183-187

[36] Kaplan PA, Tu HK, Williams SM, Lydiatt DD. The normal temporomandibular joint: MR and arthrographic correlation. Radiology. 1987;**165**:177-178

[37] Drace JE, Enzmann DR. Defining the normal temporomandibular joint: Closed-, partially open-, and open mouth MR imaging of asymptomatic subjects. Radiology. 1990;**177**:67-71

[38] Westesson PL, Eriksson L, Kurita K. Reliability of a negative clinical temporomandibular joint examination: Prevalence of disk displacement in asymptomatic temporomandibular joints. Oral Surgery, Oral Medicine, and Oral Pathology. 1989;**68**:551-554

[39] Tallents RH, Katzberg RW, Murphy W, Proskin H. Magnetic resonance imaging findings in asymptomatic volunteers and symptomatic patients with temporomandibular disorders. The Journal of Prosthetic Dentistry. 1996;**75**:529-533

[40] Katzberg RW, Westesson PL, Tallents RH, Drake CM. Anatomic disorders of the temporomandibular joint disc in asymptomatic subjects. Journal of Oral and Maxillofacial Surgery. 1996;**54**:147-153

[41] Algra PR, Bloem JL, Tissing H, et al. Detection of vertebral metastases: Comparison between MR imaging and bone scintigraphy. Radiographics. 1991;**11**:219-232

[42] Avrahami E, Tadmor R, Dally O, Hadar H. Early MR demonstration of spinal metastases in patients with normal radiographs and CT and radionuclide bone scans. Journal of Computer Assisted Tomography. 1989;**13**:598-602

[43] Jarvik JG, Deyo RA. Diagnostic evaluation of low back pain with emphasis on imaging. Annals of Internal Medicine. 2002;**137**:586-597

Adjunctive Non-surgical Aids for Management of Periodontal Problems

Oral Mesotherapy: Might Be Considered as An Adjunctive Technique for the Different Surgical Procedures?

Nermin Yussif

Abstract

The bidirectional relationship between local and systemic pathways makes it difficult to provide a safe intraoral treatment. Nowadays, mesotherapy has become more necessary in dentistry to overcome the huge number of surgical interventions either for therapeutic or for cosmetic purposes. It also limits the need for systemic drugs achieving favorable outcomes with minimal side effects. Further researches are needed to examine the usage of mesotherapy in different oral problems. In dermal mesotherapy, dermatologists used several materials as hyaluronic acid, collagen, hydroxyapatite, carboxymethyl cellulose, and silicone. Such materials exhibit different manners according to their resorption rate: temporary, semipermanent, permanent, and combinations. Furthermore, B-tricalcium phosphate and hydroxyapatite are considered as tissue stimulators by stimulation of collagen formation. Combinations of temporary materials in order to achieve immediate filling effect with tissue stimulator as HA or B-TCP achieve better results.

Keywords: oral mesotherapy, intraepidermic injection, minimally invasive techniques, vitamins, tooth traction, depigmentation, connective tissue thickening

1. An overview on the original mesotherapy technique for dermatological uses

The aim behind mesotherapy was to create a new technique, which favors the supplementation of needed agents directly and locally to the site of complaint. As previously mentioned, the proposed theory by *Pistor* depends mainly on the direct effect of the used drug on the tissue originating from the mesoderm [1, 2]. The mesoderm is one of the primary germ layers of the embryo that is responsible for the development of skin, connective tissue, muscles, tendons, and circulatory system. It is mainly responsible for skin vitality and health [3]. The injection technique of mesotherapy depends mainly on the anatomical, histological and geometrical landmarks of the target tissues. Mesointerface is the horizontal interface between the injected agents and the injected region. For maximum benefits, the injected surface is inversely proportional to the amount and molecular weight of the injected agent. The wider the mesointerface is, the greater the number of the dermal receptors that are activated [4].

On the other hand, the vertical component depends on the depth of penetration. Mesotherapy could be injected in the epidermis, dermis, or subcutaneous [1]. The more superficial injection is, the longer the drug remains in the tissue. It permits sustained release of the drug with slow and progressive diffusion into the surrounding tissues [2, 5, 6].

The technique depends on the skin characteristics and components. It determines the type of drug injected, the technique of injection, and the drug dosage. The skin has a natural sustained releasing property. Therefore, the nature of the skin determines the layers that are suitable for injection. The injection process must be in the superficial layers (intradermal) for the drug to remain as long as possible and for its clearance to become slower. If the drug is injected deeper, its clearance becomes faster. So the more superficial the injection is, the longer the drug remains in place (being far more powerful and efficient) [6].

2. FDA and mesotherapy

The FDA is the association concerning about the assurance of the food and drug safety. Although FDA did not approve the mesotherapy technique, it approved many drugs that have been used in mesotherapy as aminophylline, yohimbine, procaine, lidocaine, and marcaine [7]. Other drugs do not have the FDA approval for any purpose of usage as it is beyond the scope of FDA because they do not consider drugs as vitamins and minerals [8]. It also approved the delivery method using mesogun [1].

All the drugs used in mesotherapy are considered by the FDA as off-label used drugs. The off-label approval includes the approved drug and the approved route of administration of this drug. The local anesthetic agents calcitonin, hyaluronidase, and collagenase are not approved by the FDA [9].

3. Benefits and uses of mesotherapy

The local treatment in mesotherapy has superior advantages over the systemic one either oral or parental. Firstly, it avoids the side effects resulted from drug metabolism and excretion in the stomach, intestine, liver, and kidneys. Secondly, the effectiveness of the local drug is directly administrated into the area of interest. Finally, it minimizes the dosage used into 1% of the dosage used systemically [1].

Improvement of blood flow, removal of fibrotic tissue, an increase in the connective tissue quality and amount, hair loss (mesohair), skin rejuvenation (mesoglow), excessive fat and cellulite removal, improvement of the lymphatic drainage, osteoarthritis, and pain relief are the main medical indications of mesotherapy [10]. On the financial point of view, it is a cost-effective modality that provides successful drug delivery using inexpensive equipment with short-term practice needed for the general practitioner [11].

Oral mesotherapy is an old technique which was commonly applied in order to introduce various agents. Infiltration, intraligamentary, intramucosal, intralesional, and intraepidermic injection are common names for oral mesotherapy technique that have been used previously. The different names were more related to different layers and structures of the oral cavity.

4. Common agents delivered by oral mesotherapy

4.1 Local anesthesia

Local anesthesia is a reversible blockage of nerve conduction in a defined area that resulted in loss of sensation [12]. It can be performed using various techniques which differ according to the width of the area needed to be anesthetized as well as tissue depth and its relation to target nerve.

Local infiltration is one of the techniques in which the local anesthetic solution is administrated submucosal, intradermal, or intraligamentary in order to anesthetize the nerve endings that innervate the target region. The submucosal injection involves the drug administration in the deep dermis layer reaching the lipid layer with 45 angulation and thicker needle, while the intradermal injection involves introduction of anesthetic agent into the superficial dermis (papillary dermis) with 10 to 15 degrees using fine needle [13, 14]. Intraligamentary (or periodontal) anesthesia is a type of the locally delivered anesthetic technique in which the needle is introduced in the mesiobuccal and distobuccal directions delivering the anesthetic agent in an apical direction. Its accuracy, easiness, minimal administration of anesthetic solution, efficiency, and the lack of harmful effects to the adjacent periodontal apparatus are the main advantages of this technique [15, 16]. The pressure needed for such technique is necessary, and it remains the main cause behind the development of local inflammation and pain which may last up to 7 days as well as bone and root resorption in relation to the injection site [17]. Defective enamel disorders were also detected following intraligamentary injection of local anesthesia. In hemophilic patients, intraligamentary injections are usually not recommended to avoid hematoma formation. It was also avoided in deciduous teeth [18] (**Figure 1**).

On the other hand, the field block technique involves the introduction of the anesthetic agent in a circular configuration around the operative site [19].

The interseptal technique is a simple technique which provides adequate control of pain and bleeding especially during emergency conditions. During infection and inflammatory conditions, interseptal technique is usually preferred. A 27 gauge needle is inserted at 45° at the center of the interdental papilla. Minimal amount (0.2–0.4 ml) of the anesthetic agent is injected. It was found that interseptal technique showed higher anesthetic efficiency than the intraligamentary and intraosseous injection [18, 19].

The intrapulpal technique is one of the most common techniques that are used during endodontic treatment especially in acute phases of pulpal inflammation.

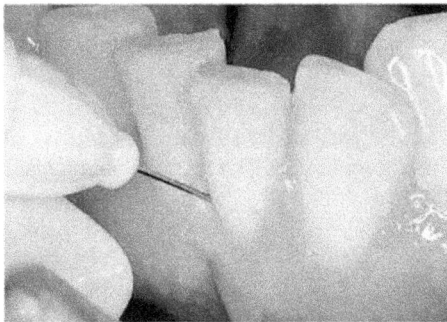

Figure 1.
Intraligamentary injection [18].

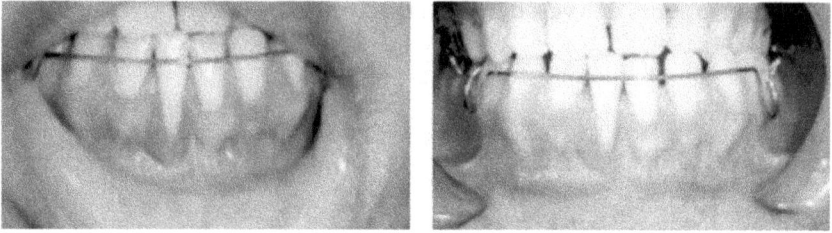

Figure 2.
Corticosteroids and chronic gingival inflammation.

Despite its rapid onset, effectiveness, and safeness, its action has shorter duration than other techniques [18]. Finally, the intraosseous technique provides rapid introduction, which is commonly used following failure of the field or nerve block technique. It depends on the direct introduction of the anesthetic agent to the interdental bone resulting in rapid delivery of the anesthetic agent to the blood circulation which should be avoided in cardiovascular patients [19] (**Figure 2**).

4.2 Corticosteroids

Corticosteroids are widely used for the management of numerous oral inflammatory conditions due to their anti-inflammatory and immune modulatory effects. They could be delivered either intramucosally (within the lesion), topically, or systemically [20].

Intralesional (intradermal) corticosteroid injection is a favorite method in delivering the drug directly to the target site resulting in rapid action as well as less systemic complications. Injectable steroids are clear fluids; their color and dose depend on the formulation of steroids used. It is commonly used in managing the longstanding oral lichen planus lesions and oral submucous fibrosis, but it has a localized side effect such as mucosal atrophy [21, 22]. Hydrocortisone and triamcinolone are the commonest formulas used in local delivery with weekly injections reaching up to 11 injections [22, 23].

Although surgical excision is considered the gold standard technique for treating mucocele and orofacial granulomatosis, the use of intralesional corticosteroid injection was also reported. However, some investigators have suggested that the intralesional corticosteroid could be used as a new modality in the treatment, but cases of relapse with corticosteroid have been reported [24, 25]. Great differences were detected in the used doses and the number of sessions according to the severity, extension, and the systemic condition of the patient [22, 23, 26–28].

4.3 Vitamins

According to literature, vitamins were usually introduced either by intraligamentary or intraepidermic techniques. The intraepidermic technique was conducted in 2016 by Yussif et al. [29].

4.3.1 Vitamin D

Although vitamin D has a great role in maintaining the bone health and metabolism, it is just recently discovered that vitamin D deficiency has a great role in the occurrence and progression of various periodontal diseases. It is a steroid hormone that controls the bone metabolism and calcium homeostasis [30–32].

It was detected that the level of vitamin D reaches its lowest levels during periodontal disease especially aggressive periodontitis. The daily supplementation is important to maintain the periodontal health [30–33].

The introduction of locally delivered vitamin D injections provides short treatment visits, non-traumatic, less patient morbidity, non-stressful procedure with no post-operative side effects. The procedure is not painful. There is also no need for preoperative local anesthesia. It could be either delivered alone [34] or in combination with calcium [35]. The promising improvement of the regenerative power was attributed to minimal trauma and preserving the periosteum adapted over the alveolar bone. Great reduction of the clinical attachment loss and the absence of bleeding on probing were also detected indicating the absence of inflammation. On the radiographic examination, improvement of the alveolar bone density as well as accentuation of lamina dura was also reported [34, 35].

In orthodontic therapy, locally delivered vitamin D is commonly introduced in small doses using periodontal injection technique in order to accelerate the osteoclastic activity in the pressure site which in role accelerates the orthodontic movement. The dose and the number of the treatment sessions are determined according to the distance that the tooth needed to travel [34, 36] (**Figure 3**).

4.3.2 Vitamin C

Ascorbic acid is also an essential vitamin in the treatment of periodontal diseases. Its deficiency causes impaired wound healing with higher bleeding index. Lower levels of serum vitamin C were reported in periodontitis. The importance of vitamin C lies behind its powerful scavenging and antioxidant effect as it usually

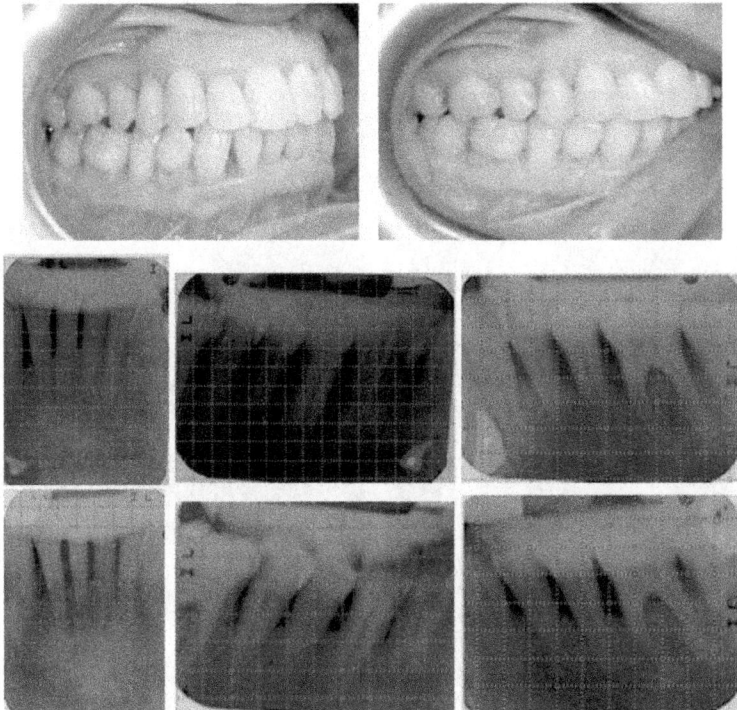

Figure 3.
Vitamin D injection and periodontitis [37].

accumulates in the immune cells as PMNs and macrophages and significantly enhances chemotaxis, phagocytic, opsonization, degranulation, and killing functions of immune cells [33, 38]. It also has a great role in collagen biosynthesis [39]. It could be supplied orally, topically, or by intraepidermal injection [37, 40]. Vitamin C is widely used in dermal mesotherapy as it restores the tissue integrity and brightness by neutralizing the free radicals in the newly formed tissues, stimulates the collagen formation, and inhibits melanogenesis [10, 41].

Growing evidence has suggested the role of vitamin C in enhancing the quality and outcome of the orthodontic treatment. This is proven when tooth movement was enhanced following systemic administration of vitamin C for 17 days [42, 43]. It was also noticed that its deficiency is accompanied with limited tooth movement and arrested osteogenesis [44].

Vitamin C induces its action through modifying the osteoclastic activity, osteogenesis, tissue healing, and periodontal ligament organization. It increases the collagen I synthesis that represents the main component of bone matrix and periodontal ligament [45]. It also accelerates the bone mineralization, calcium absorption, formation of collagen type X, expression of alkaline phosphatase, and osteoblast growth and differentiation [46, 47] (**Figure 4**).

Furthermore, the depigmenting effect of vitamin C depends mainly on its antioxidant property. The efficiency of vitamin C in the treatment of physiologic or pathologic dermal problems such as hyperpigmentation, aging, and dryness was promising due to several factors that are not only related to its direct interaction with melanin and melanocytes but also due to the overall effect on the applied tissues. Once vitamin C is introduced to the target tissue, it binds efficiently to melanin because melanin is the main store of ROS, calcium, and copper content that causes intracellular deficiency of these items. Lower intracellular calcium level causes failure of melanocytes to perform cellular adhesion as calcium is essential to form cadherins [48, 49]. The contact to keratinocytes is important simulator to

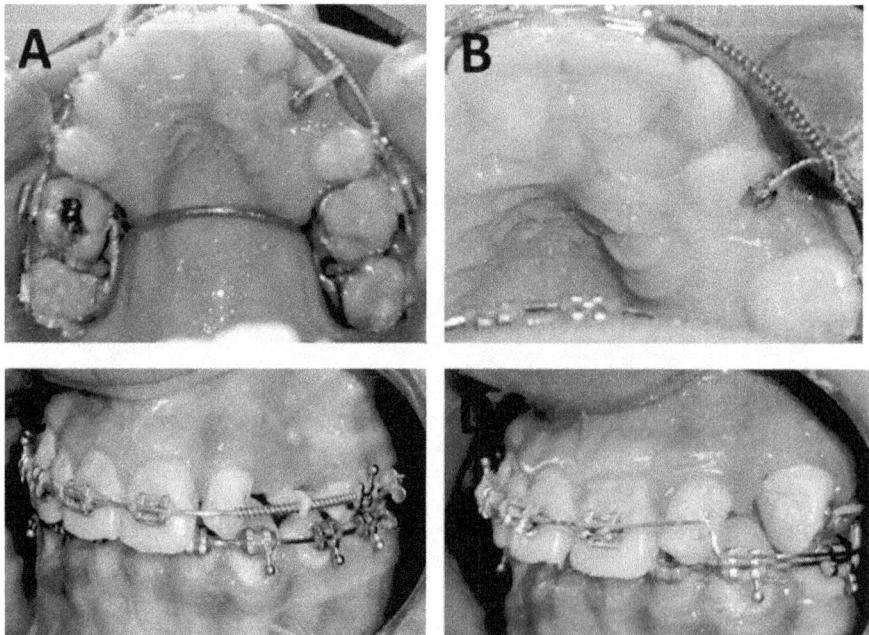

Figure 4.
Pre- and postoperative local vitamin C injection in impacted canine traction [37].

melanocytes to produce melanin, formation of dendrites and transfer the produced melanin to neighboring cells [48, 50]. Also, shortage of the intercellular copper limits the formation of tyrosine, tyrosinase enzyme, and peroxidase enzyme which in turn stops the melanin production [41].

Pain and itching were regarded as painful stimuli. Itching may transit to pain due to increased discharge frequency of nociceptors (intensity theory) [51] (**Figure 5**).

In 2016, Yussif et al. used the intraepidermic injection technique (oral mesotherapy technique) in order to treat physiological hyperpigmentation. Vitamin C injection is a safe, minimally invasive nonsurgical depigmenting technique which also improves health of gingival tissues. They concluded that the direct effect of vitamin C could be due to the affinity of melanin to react with it, which in turn affects the cellular junctions (causing the immediate fainting) and forces such cells to spell out their contents of melanin leading to tissue darkening after a while. Further investigations and studies are recommended to detect its long-term effect on the melanocytes and keratinocytes [29] (**Figure 6**).

During persistent gingival inflammation, Yussif et al. [45] have reported significant enhancement of the gingival health by the usage of the intraepidermic vitamin C injection as an adjunctive approach for the conventional nonsurgical treatment modality.

During inflammation, it was found that the tissue antioxidant level (as vitamin C, vitamin E, etc.) decreases rapidly indicating the need of its supplementation. On the other hand, the free radical production increases at the site of inflammation [52, 53]. Extra doses of antioxidants especially vitamin C are essential. In localized inflammatory conditions, the administration of the needed higher doses via systemic route (higher than 500 mg) cannot be absorbed by the gastrointestinal tract, which is easily excreted through urine. Moreover, in order to reach this dose at the site of inflammation, it needs administration of very high systemic doses that could be harmful to the patient. The local injection provides the needed dose efficiently [54] (**Figure 7**).

In 2014, [55] reported that the switch of the gingival tissue to the thick biotype is important to gingival and periodontal health as well as esthetic outcome. Ascorbic acid enhances the periodontal ligament maturation and renewal by induction of the collagen formation especially collagen III (young collagen) and keeps the balance between collagen I (mature collagen) and III for tissue maturation. It also modifies the rate of fibroblast proliferation [56]. In 2016, Yussif et al. reported the improvement of the gingival biotype following the intraepidermic vitamin C injection ranging between 0.5 and 1 mm [29].

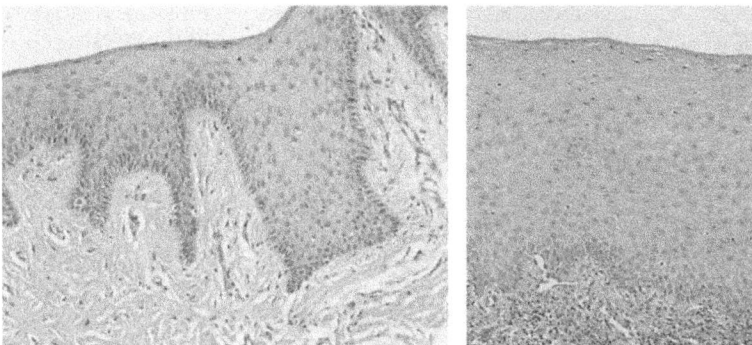

Figure 5.
Pre- and postoperative histopathological photos of local vitamin C injection in treatment of gingival hyperpigmentation [29].

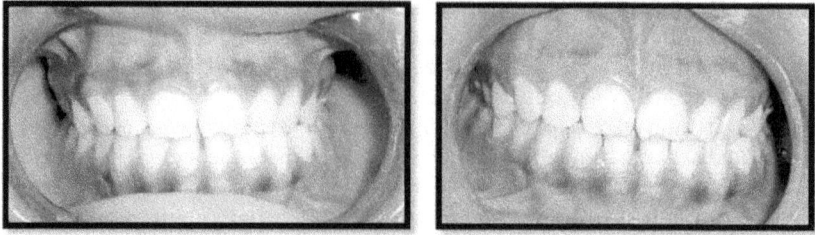

Figure 6.
Pre- and postoperative local vitamin C injection in physiologic gingival hyperpigmentation [29].

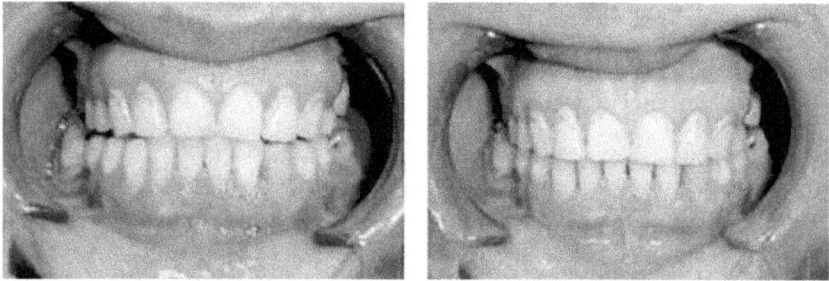

Figure 7.
Pre- and postoperative local vitamin C injection in gingival inflammation [45].

4.4 Autogenous blood products

Platelet-rich plasma (PRP) is defined as a portion of the plasma element of autologous blood having a platelet concentration above baseline [56, 57]. It is considered as a growth factor agonist [58] with both mitogenic and chemotactic properties [56].

It was found that intralesional injection is a newly described method for application of PRP and represents an effective therapeutic option when dealing with non-healing wounds [59]. These findings open the door for using intralesional PRP in oral chronic ulcers. In 2015, El-Komy and his colleagues conducted a pilot study on seven patients suffering from resistant chronic oral pemphigus vulgaris (PV). All patients reported improvement in pain scores, ability to eat, and healing score [60].

In orthodontic therapy, significant improvement was reported following the introduction of local submucosal PRP injection in the pressure side. A single injection of PRP was enough during active orthodontic treatment (just 2 injections; pre and after 6 months). Acceleration of orthodontic tooth movement was reported 1.7-fold when compared to the conventional traction technique [61] (**Figure 8**).

4.5 Hyaluronic acid

Black triangles or insufficient interdental papillae are considered a serious esthetic problem especially in patients with high lip line [62, 63].

Hyaluronic acid is an important component of the extracellular matrix, which has great role in maintaining the health of the oral tissues and healing and repair process. The mechanism of its action depends mainly on stimulating the cellular proliferation, migration, and vasculature and restoring the integrity of epidermal and dermal layer. It is also effective in stimulating collagen formation through enhancing the proliferation of fibroblasts. In dentistry, it is recently used

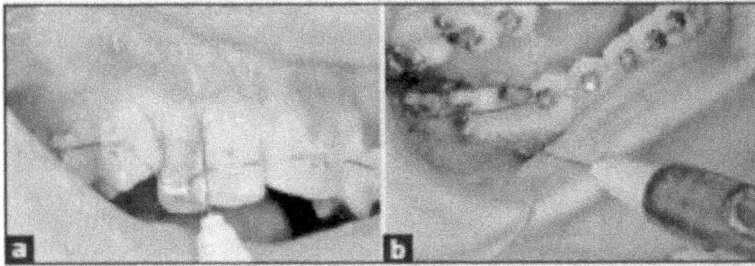

Figure 8.
Submucosal injection of PRP during orthodontic treatment [61].

to accelerate the healing of oral ulcers [64], extraction socket [65], and gingival inflammation [66] either through injection or topical application. It was also used in reconstruction of the interdental papilla as a minimally invasive technique instead of the conventional surgical intervention [67, 68].

4.6 Parathyroid hormone injection

Parathyroid hormone is one of the essential hormones that affect the bone metabolism. It was found that its local injection provides acceleration of the orthodontic tooth movement 1.6 times faster than the normal movement range. A daily local injection of parathyroid hormone (PTH) was also used to induce local bone resorption by reducing the concentration of the gel medium using saline [69, 70].

4.7 Relaxin hormone injection

Relaxin is a specialized hormone which was detected in the periodontal ligament providing proper remodeling of the soft tissue rather than the alveolar bone surrounding teeth. It provides the needed balance of the collagen content in the pressure and tension sites especially during application of forces as orthodontic treatment. It was found that the local injection of relaxin could provide an accelerated tooth movement by reducing the organization of the related periodontal ligaments and increasing the tooth mobility. A weekly injection of 50 μg of relaxin hormone was also found to accelerate tooth movement via soft tissue remodeling, rather than bone, through increasing the collagen at the tension side over its amount in the compression side. It also decreases the organization of the periodontal ligaments surrounding the tooth causing extra mobility [70–72].

4.8 Prostaglandin injection

Prostaglandin is one of the most important inflammatory mediators that is usually secreted during the inflammatory process. It is also considered as a paracrine hormone which affects mainly bone resorption level around the teeth by affecting the osteoclastic activity. It was found that its local application provides 1.6-fold of accelerated tooth movement than the normal range. Formerly, exogenous single or multiple prostaglandin injections were used [70, 73, 74].

4.9 Simvastatin

Simvastatin is a chemical agent that is usually used to reduce the serum cholesterol level. It was found that it has a positive, stimulatory effect to the bone by stimulation of bone growth factors (e.g., BMP-2). On local injection, it was found that simvastatin could efficiently treat the infrabony defects and furcation defects and be used for guided bone regeneration. The injection visits could range from one to three times with 0.5–2 ml per visit. It is considered a successful nonsurgical treatment approach [75] (**Figure 9**).

4.10 Bone morphogenic proteins (BMPs)

In orthopedics, recombinant BMPs were commonly used during distraction of long bones in order to accelerate osteogenic potentials, increase bone volume (both width and height), improve bone density, and reduce relapse possibilities. BMP-2 was commonly used with or without delivery systems as collagen sponge and chitosan hydrogel in sequential injections [75, 76] (**Figure 10**).

4.11 Combinations

Hyaluronidase is one of the proteolytic enzymes that are providing a physiologic limiting factor for intercellular cement substance, hyaluronic acid. It was used in the treatment of submucous fibrosis by promoting the lysis of accumulated fibrous tissues and relieving the stiffness of tissues by intralesional injection. It provides a rapid short-term improvement [29, 78]. In addition, corticosteroids could be combined with bisphosphonates in the treatment of central giant cell lesions with neither recurrence nor clinical side effects being detected [27].

Steroids are well-known immunosuppressive agents which offer a control of the inflammation. Up till now, different types of cortisone were used to undergo the needed outcome as triamcinolone and dexamethasone. Despite its potency, it was preferred because of its cost-effectiveness. Single-dose injection per week was needed till improvement is detected, which may extend to 4 months. Progression could be detected after two injections [29, 77].

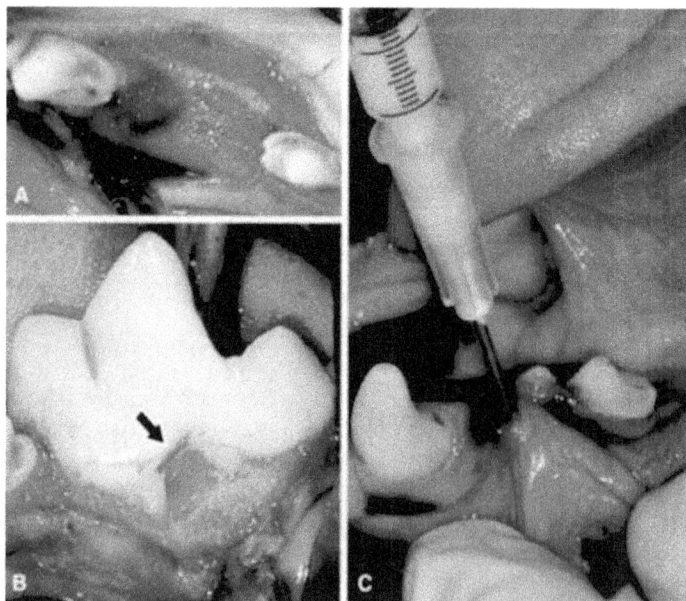

Figure 9.
Simvastatin injection [75].

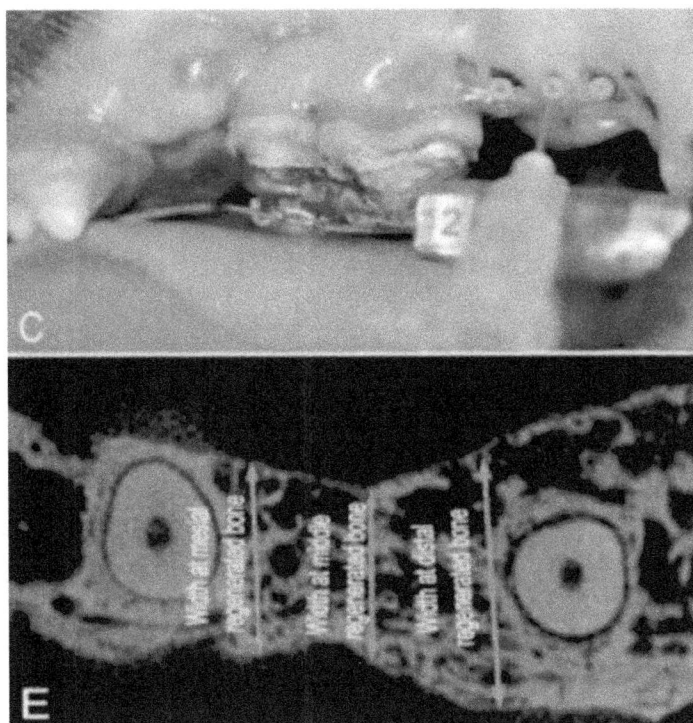

Figure 10.
Bone morphogenic protein injection [75].

The usage of hyaluronidase and cortisone injection combination provides long-term improvement of the signs and symptoms associated with such diseases, bringing sensation, ulceration, and pain [29, 77].

5. Oral mesotherapy injection protocol

According to literature, up till now there is no definite protocol for dermal mesotherapy. In the oral cavity, it was more difficult to add specific rules due to the presence of multiple geometry, types, and dimensions of tissues as gingiva, buccal mucosa, palate, tongue, etc.; we have tried to establish guidelines for general practitioners and beginners.

- Oral mesotherapy technique needs longer time for practice in order to achieve better results.

- Only minute quantities of injectable agent ranging between 0.05 and 0.1 ml/point are permissible according to the range of the injected tissue expansion.

- In 1965, *Woodard* recommended that the pH of any injected material should range between 4.5 and 8.0. Local injections show lower rate of buffering capacity than intravenous and intramuscular route. During oral mesotherapy injection, higher pH is preferred.

- The used needle has to be short, beveled. The needle's gauge should range between 25 and 30.

- Numerous sites for administration of different injectable products are still acceptable till now. The buccal mucosa, buccal vestibule, palate, labial gingival tissues, interdental papilla, and tongue are the most common sites for local injections.

- On the contrary to the skin, oral mucosa is always wet. Surface cleaning and dryness using dry gauze is recommended without the usage of surface disinfectant. Local anesthetic or analgesic agent (specific for intraoral usage) is also recommended accompanying the usage of specific agents as vitamin C due to its nature as a weak acid. In general, the usage of any injectable agent causes local inflammation and induces pain and itching.

- Preoperative treatment plan and patient preparation are the most important steps in the whole treatment procedure. Detailed patient's medical history is an important issue. The target tissue should be free of infection and clean. Two visits for periodontal debridement are recommended; the first is preferred to be performed 2 weeks prior to the procedure, while the other is usually performed prior to the injection visit especially if the injection will be more related to the teeth. The patient should be instructed to keep away from vitamin E and aspirin 1 week before the injection session. After the session, the patient must be instructed that discomfort or burning could occur for 20 minutes. Analgesics are not permitted.

6. Complications and criticism of mesotherapy

The main complications reported in this technique include ulceration, bleeding, infections, allergy, abscess, hyperpigmentation, and swelling related to the area to be injected [78, 79]. The main problems of mesotherapy are the lack of training of the practitioner, the difficulty to be evaluated except with biopsy, the inability to diagnose and treat a complication, and the lack of standardized dosage or formulation [1].

Author details

Nermin Yussif[1,2,3]

1 NILES, Cairo University, Cairo, Egypt

2 Periodontology Department, Faculty of Dentistry, Cairo University, Cairo, Egypt

3 Periodontology Department, Faculty of Dentistry, MSA University, Giza, Egypt

*Address all correspondence to: dr_nermin_yusuf@yahoo.com

IntechOpen

References

[1] Materasso A, Pfeifar T. Mesotherapy for body contouring. Plastic and Reconstructive Surgery. 2005;**115**:1420-1424

[2] Mammucari M, Gatti A, Maggiori S, Bartoletti C, Sabato A. Mesotherapy, definition, rationale and clinical role: A consensus report from the Italian society of mesotherapy. European Review for Medical and Pharmacological Sciences. 2011;**15**:682-694

[3] Adelson H. French mesotherapy for the treatment of pain. Bulletin SFM. 2006;**4**:57

[4] Herreros F, de Moraes A, Velho P. Mesotherapy: A bibliographical review. Anais Brasileiros de Dermatologia. 2011;**86**(1):96-101

[5] Binaglia L, Marconi P, Pitzurra M. The diffusion of intradermally administered procaine. Journal of Mesotherapy. 1981;**1**:15-28

[6] American Society of Plastic Surgeons (ASPS) guiding principles for mesotherapy. 2008;7(8)

[7] Menkes C et al. Controlled trial of injectable diclofenac in mesotherapy for the treatment of tendinitis. Bulletin SFM. 2002;**4**:250-252

[8] Palermo S et al. Mesotherapy association in the therapy of cervicobrachialgia. Minerva Anestesiologica. 1991;**57**:1084-1085

[9] Rutunda A, Kolodney M. Mesotherapy and phosphatidylcholine injections: Historical clarification and review. Dermatologic Surgery. 2006;**32**:465

[10] Bryant R. Aloe vera: Nature's soothing healer to periodontal disease - controversial mesotherapy. Dermatology Times. 2004;**25**(1):4-8

[11] Sivagnanam G. Mesotherapy—The French connection. 2010;**1**(1):4-8

[12] Achar S, Kundu S. Principles of office anesthesia: Part I. Infiltrative anesthesia. American Family Physician. 2002;**66**(1):91-94

[13] McGee D. Local and topical anesthesia. In: Roberts JR, Hedges J, editors. Clinical Procedures in Emergency Medicine. 4th ed. Philadelphia, PA: WB Saunders; 2004. pp. 533-551

[14] Heavner J. Local anesthetics. Current Opinion in Anaesthesiology. 2007;**20**(4):336-342

[15] Tsirlis A, Iakovidis D, Parisis N. Dry socket: Frequency of occurrence after intra-ligamentary anesthesia. Quintessence International. 1992;**23**(8):575-577

[16] Meechan J, Thomason J. A comparison of 2 topical anesthetics on the discomfort of intraligamentary injections: A double-blind, split-mouth volunteers clinical trial. Oral Surgery, Oral Medicine, Oral Pathology, and Oral Radiology. 1999;**87**(3):62-65

[17] Lalabonova P, Kirova D, Dobreva D. Intraligamentary anesthesia in general dental practice. Hristina Journal of IMAB—Annual Proceeding. 2005;**11**:22-24

[18] Gazal G, Fareed W, Zafar M. Role of intraseptal anesthesia for pain-free dental treatment. Saudi Journal of Anesthesia. 2010;**10**(1):81-86

[19] Tom K, Aps J. Intraosseous anesthesia as a primary technique for local anesthesia in dentistry. Clinical Research in Infectious Diseases. 2015;**2**(1):1012

[20] Masthan K, Aravindha BN, Jha A, Elumalai M. Steroids application inoral

diseases. International Journal of Pharma and Bio Sciences. 2013;**4**: 829-834

[21] Xia J, Li C, Hong Y, Yang L, Huang Y, Cheng B. Short-term clinical evaluation of intralesional triamcinolone acetonide injection for ulcerative oral lichen planus. Journal of Oral Pathology and Medicine. 2006;**35**(6):327-331

[22] Singh M, Niranjan H, Mehrotra R, Sharma D, Gupta S. Efficacy of hydrocortisone acetate/hyaluronidase vs triamcinolone acetonide/hyaluronidase in the treatment of oral submucous fibrosis. The Indian Journal of Medical Research. 2010;**131**:665-669

[23] Schlosser B. Lichen planus and lichenoid reactions of the oral mucosa. Dermatologic Therapy. 2010;**23**:251-267

[24] Baharvand M, Sabounchi S, Mortazavi H. Treatment of labial mucocele by intralesional injection of dexamethasone: Case series. 2014;**3**:128-133

[25] Javali M, Tapashetti R, Deshmukh J. Esthetic management of gingival hyperpigmentation: Report of two cases. International Journal of Dental Clinics. 2011;**3**(2):115-116

[26] da Silva NG, Carreira S, Pedreira E, Tuji F, Ortega K, Pinheiro J. Treatment of central giant cell lesions using bisphosphonates with intralesional corticosteroid injections. Head and Face Medicine. 2012;**8**:23

[27] Fedele S, Fung P, Bamashmous N, Petrie A, Porter S. Long-term effectiveness of intralesional triamcinolone acetonide therapy in orofacial granulomatosis: An observational cohort study. 2014:794-801

[28] Goswami R, Gangwani A, Bhatnagar S, Singh D. Comparative study of oral nutritional supplements vs intralesional triamcinolone and hyaluronidase in oral submucous fibrosis. International Journal of Medical Research and Review. 2014;**2**(2):114-118

[29] Yussif N, Zayed S, Hasan S, Sadek S. Evaluation of injectable vitamin C as a depigmenting agent in physiologic gingival melanin hyperpigmentation: A clinical trial. 2016;**8**(6):113-120

[30] Amano Y, Komiyama K, Makishima M. Vitamin D and periodontal disease. Journal of Oral Science. 2009;**51**(1):11-20

[31] Liu K, Meng H, Lu R, Xu L, Zhang L, Chen Z, et al. Initial periodontal therapy reduced systemic and local 25-hydroxy vitamin D3 and interleukin-1b in patients with aggressive periodontitis periodontal inflammation. Journal of Periodontology. 2010;**81**:260-266

[32] Zhang X, Meng H, Xu L, Zhang L, Shi D, Feng X, et al. Vitamin D-binding protein levels in plasma and gingival crevicular fluid of patients with generalized aggressive periodontitis. International Journal of Endocrinology. 2014;**783575**:1-6

[33] Van der Velden U, Kuzmanova D, Chapple I. Micronutritional approaches to periodontal therapy. Journal of Clinical Periodontology. 2011;**38**(11):142-158

[34] Al-Hasani N, Al-Bustani A, Ghareeb M, Hussain S. Clinical efficacy of locally injected calcitriol in orthodontic tooth movement. International Journal of Pharmacy and Pharmaceutical Sciences. 2011;**3**(5):139-143

[35] Yussif N, Korany N, Abbass M. Evidence of the effect of intraepidermic vitamin C injection on melanocytes and keratinocytes in gingival tissues: In vivo study. Dentistry. 2017;**7**(3):2-6

[36] Collins M, Sinclair P. The local use- of vitamin D to increase the rate of orthodontic tooth movement. American Journal of Orthodontics and Dentofacial Orthopedics. 1988;**94**:278-284

[37] Yussif NM, El-Mahdi FM, Wagih R. Hypothyroidism as a risk factor of periodontitis and its relation with vitamin D deficiency: Mini-review of literature and a case report. Clinical Cases in Mineral and Bone Metabolism. 2017;**14**(3):312-316

[38] Kuzmanova D, Jansen I, Schoenmaker T, Nazmi K, Teeuw W, Bizzarro S, et al. Vitamin C in plasma and leucocytes in relation to periodontitis. Journal of Clinical Periodontology. 2012;**39**:905-912

[39] Padayatty S, Katz A, Wang Y, Eck P, Kwon O, Lee J, et al. Vitamin C as an antioxidant: Evaluation of its role in disease prevention. Journal of the American College of Nutrition. 2003;**22**(1):18-35

[40] Shimada Y, Tai H, Tanaka A, Ikezawa-Suzuki I, Takagi K, Yoshida Y, et al. Effects of ascorbic acid on gingival melanin pigmentation in vitro and in vivo. Journal of Periodontology. 2009;**80**:317-323

[41] Chase C. Common complications and adverse reactions. Bulletin SFM. 2005;**10**(8)

[42] Strause L, Saltman P, Glowacki J. The effect of deficiencies of manganese and copper on osteoinduction and on resorption of bone particles in rats. Calcified Tissue International. 1987;**41**(3):145-150

[43] De Laurenzi V, Melino G, Savini I, Annicchiarico-Petruzzelli M, Finazzi-Agrò A, Avigliano L. Cell death by oxidative stress and ascorbic acid regeneration in human neuroectodermal cell

lines. European Journal of Cancer. 1995;**31A**(4):463-466

[44] Miresmaeili A, Mollaei N, Azar R, Farhadian N, Kashani K. Effect of dietary vitamin C on orthodontic tooth movement in rats. Journal of Dentistry. 2015;**12**(6):409-413

[45] Yussif N, Abdul AM, Abdel RA. Evaluation of the anti-inflammatory effect of locally delivered vitamin C in the treatment of persistent gingival inflammation: Clinical and histopathological study. Journal of Nutrition and Metabolism. 2016;**2978741**:1-8

[46] Aghajanian P, Hall S, Wongworawat M, Mohan S. The roles and mechanisms of actions of vitamin C in bone: New developments. Journal of Bone and Mineral Research. 2015;**30**(11):1945-1955

[47] Jokar A, Farahi F, Asadi N, Salehi M, Foruhari S, Sayadi M. The effect of vitamin C on bone mineral/mass density of menopausal women with equilibrated regime: A randomized clinical trial. Biomedical Research. 2015;**26**(2):239-244

[48] Kippenberger S, Bernd A, Bereiter-Hahn J, Amirez-Bosca A, Kaufmann R. The mechanism of melanocyte dendrite formation: The impact of differentiating keratinocytes. Pigment Cell Research. 1998;**11**:34-37

[49] Tolleson W. Human melanocyte biology, toxicology and pathology. Journal of Environmental Science and Health. 2005;**23**:105-161

[50] Letort V, Fouliard S, Letort G, Adanja I, Kumasaka M, Gallagher S, et al. Quantitative analysis of melanocyte migration in vitro based on automated cell tracking under phase contrast microscopy considering the combined influence of cell division and cell-matrix interactions. Mathematical

Modelling of Natural Phenomena, EDP Sciences. 2010;5(1):4-33

[51] Schmelz M. Translating nociceptive processing into human pain models. Experimental Brain Research. 2009;196(1):173-178

[52] Mohammed BM, Fisher BJ, Huynh QK, et al. Resolution of sterile inflammation: Role for vitamin C. Mediators of Inflammation. 2014;2014:Article ID:173403

[53] Daniels A, Jefferies S. Analysis of capacity of novel, anti-oxidant tooth paste, small population clinical study: Comparison to levels of gingival inflammation reduction reported in historical control and therapeutic tooth brushing studies. 2003

[54] Shimabukuro Y, Nakayama Y, Ogata Y, Tamazawa K, Shimauchi H, Nishida T, et al. Effects of an ascorbic acid derivative dentifrices in patients with gingivitis: A double masked, randomized, controlled clinical trial. Journal of Periodontology. 2015;86:27-35

[55] Abraham S, Deepak K, Ambili R, Preeja C, Archana V. Gingival biotype and its clinical significance: A review. The Saudi Journal for Dental Research. 2014;5:3-7

[56] Marx R. Platelet-rich plasma (PRP): What is PRP and what is not PRP? Implant Dentistry. 2001;10:225-228

[57] Mehta S, Watson J. Platelet rich concentrate: Basic science and current clinical applications. Journal of Orthopaedic Trauma. 2008;22:432-438

[58] Petrova N, Edmonds M. Emerging drugs for diabetic foot ulcers. Expert Opinion on Emerging Drugs. 2006;11:709-724

[59] Wasterlain AS, Braun HJ, Harris AH, Kim HJ, Dragoo JL. The systemic effects of platelet-rich plasma injection. American Journal of Sports Medicine. 2013;41(1):186-193. DOI: 10.1177/0363546512466383. Epub 2012 Dec 4

[60] El-Komy M, Hassan A, Raheem H, Doss S, El-Kaliouby M, Saleh N, et al. Platelet-rich plasma for resistant oral erosions of *Pemphigus vulgaris*: A pilot study. Wound Repair and Regeneration. 2015;23:953-955

[61] Liou E. The development of submucosal injection of platelet rich plasma for accelerating orthodontic tooth movement and preserving pressure side alveolar bone. APOS Trends in Orthodontics. 2016;6:5-11

[62] McGuire MK, Scheyer ET. A randomized, double-blind, placebo-controlled study to determine the safety and efficacy of cultured and expanded autologous fibroblast injections for the treatment of interdental papillary insufficiency associated with the papilla priming procedure. Journal of Periodontology. 2007;78(1):4-17

[63] Mansouri S, Ghasemi M, Salmani Z, Shams N. Clinical application of hyaluronic acid gel for reconstruction of interdental papilla at the esthetic zone. The Journal of Islamic Dental Association of IRAN (JIDA). 2013;25(2):191-196

[64] Nolon A, Baillie C, Badminton J, Rudralinglam M, Seymour R. The efficacy of topical hyaluronic acid in the management of recurrent aphthous ulceration. Journal of Oral Pathology and Medicine. 2006;35(8):461-465

[65] Mendes R, Silva G, Lima M, Calliari M, Almeida A, Alves J, et al. Sodium hyaluronate accelerates the healing process in tooth sockets of rats. Archives of Oral Biology. 2008;53(12):1155-1162

[66] Jentsch H, Pomowski R, Kundt G, Göcke R. Treatment of gingivitis with hyaluronan. The Journal of Clinical Periodontology. 2003;**30**(2):159-164

[67] Becker W, Gabitov I, Stepanov M, Kois J, Smidt A, Becker B. Minimally invasive treatment for papillae deficiencies in the esthetic zone: A pilot study. Clinical Implant Dentistry and Related Research. 2010;**12**(1):1-8

[68] Mansouri SS, Ghasemi M, Salmani Z, Shams N. Clinical application of hyaluronic acid gel for reconstruction of interdental papilla at the esthetic zone. Journal of Islamic Dental Association of Iran. 2013;**25**:152-157

[69] Soma S, Matsumoto S, Higuchi Y, Takano-Yamamoto T, Yamashita K, Kurisu K, et al. Local and chronic application of PTH accelerates tooth movement in rats. Journal of Dental Research. 2000;**79**(9):1717-1724

[70] Nimeri G, Kau C, Abou-Kheir N, Corona R. Acceleration of tooth movement during orthodontic treatment—A frontier in orthodontics. Progress in Orthodontics. 2013;**14**:42

[71] Liu Z, King G, Gu G, Shin J, Stewart D. Does human relaxin accelerate orthodontic tooth movement in rats? Annals of the New York Academy of Sciences. 2005;**1041**:388-394

[72] McGorray S, Dolce C, Kramer S, Stewart D, Wheeler T. A randomized, placebo-controlled clinical trial on the effects of recombinant human relaxin on tooth movement and short-term stability. American Journal of Orthodontics and Dentofacial Orthopedics. 2012;**141**(2):196-203

[73] Yamasaki K, Shibata Y, Imai S, Tani Y, Shibasaki Y, Fukuhara T. Clinical application of prostaglandin E1 (PGE1)

upon orthodontic tooth movement. American Journal of Orthodontics. 1984;**85**(6):508-518

[74] Seifi M, Eslami B, Saffar AS. The effect of prostaglandin E2 and calcium gluconate on orthodontic tooth movement and root resorption in rats. European Journal of Orthodontics. 2003;**25**(2):199-204

[75] Morris M, Lee Y, Lavin MT, Giannini PJ, Schmid MJ, Marx DB, et al. Injectable simvastatin in periodontal defects and alveolar ridges: Pilot studies. Journal of Periodontology. 2008;**79**:1465-1473

[76] Terbish M, Yoo S, Kim H, Yu H, Hwang C, Baik H, et al. Accelerated bone formation in distracted alveolar bone after injection of recombinant human bone morphogenetic protein-2. Journal of Periodontology. 2015;**86**:1078-1086

[77] James L, Shetty A, Rishi D, Abraham M. Management of oral submucous fibrosis with injection of hyaluronidase and dexamethasone in grade III oral submucous fibrosis: A retrospective study. Journal of International Oral Health. 2015;7(8):1-4

[78] Davis M, Wright T, Shehan J. A complication of mesotherapy: Noninfectious granulomatous panniculitis. Archives of Dermatology. 2008;**144**:808

[79] Conforti G, Capone L, Corra S. Intradermal therapy (mesotherapy) for the treatment of acute pain in carpal tunnel syndrome: A preliminary study. The Korean Journal of Pain. 2014;**27**(1):49-53